THE LIBRARY
North Devon District Hospital
Raleigh Park, Barnstaple
Devon EX31 4JB
Tel: 01271 - 322363
rary@ndevon.swest.nhs.uk

~ t' ~t date stamped '

Withdrawn	
Reason:	
Date:	
By:	

Question Everything

ocket tutor

D1387361

Psychiatry

Tomasz Bajorek BA Hons (Oxon) BM BCh
Core Trainee in Psychiatry
Warneford Hospital
Oxford, UK

Thomas Stockmann MA (Oxon) BM BCh
Core Trainee in Psychiatry
Homerton Hospital
London, UK

Editorial Advisor

Neel Burton BSc MBBS MRCPsych MA (Phil) AKC
Tutor in Psychiatry
Green Templeton College
University of Oxford
Oxford, UK

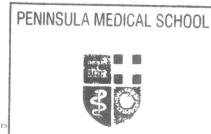

PENINSULA MEDICAL SCHOOL

JP
medical
publishers

© 2012 JP Medical Ltd.

Published by JP Medical Ltd, 83 Victoria Street, London, SW1H 0HW, UK

Tel: +44 (0)20 3170 8910 Fax: +44 (0)20 3008 6180

Email: info@jpmedpub.com Web: www.jpmedpub.com

The rights of Tomasz Bajorek and Thomas Stockmann to be identified as the authors of this work have been asserted by them in accordance with the Copyright, Designs and Patents Act 1988.

All rights reserved. No part of this publication may be reproduced, stored or transmitted in any form or by any means, electronic, mechanical, photocopying, recording or otherwise, except as permitted by the UK Copyright, Designs and Patents Act 1988, without the prior permission in writing of the publishers. Permissions may be sought directly from JP Medical Ltd at the address printed above.

All brand names and product names used in this book are trade names, service marks, trademarks or registered trademarks of their respective owners. The publisher is not associated with any product or vendor mentioned in this book.

Medical knowledge and practice change constantly. This book is designed to provide accurate, authoritative information about the subject matter in question. However, readers are advised to check the most current information available on procedures included or from the manufacturer of each product to be administered, to verify the recommended dose, formula, method and duration of administration, adverse effects and contraindications. It is the responsibility of the practitioner to take all appropriate safety precautions. Neither the publisher nor the authors assume any liability for any injury and/or damage to persons or property arising from or related to use of the material in this book.

This book is sold on the understanding that the publisher is not engaged in providing professional medical services. If such advice or services are required, the services of a competent medical professional should be sought.

ISBN: 978-1-907816-23-9

British Library Cataloguing in Publication Data
A catalogue record for this book is available from the British Library

Library of Congress Cataloging in Publication Data
A catalog record for this book is available from the Library of Congress

JP Medical Ltd is a subsidiary of Jaypee Brothers Medical Publishers (P) Ltd, New Delhi, India.

Publisher:	Richard Furn
Development Editor:	Paul Mayhew
Editorial Assistant:	Katrina Rimmer
Design:	Designers Collective Ltd
Index:	Liz Granger

Typeset, printed and bound in India.

Foreword

He said the soul was treated with certain charms, my dear Charmides, and that these charms were beautiful words.
   Plato (d. 347-8 BC), *Charmides*

'Psychiatry' derives from the Ancient Greek and literally means 'healing of the soul'. In one of Plato's early dialogues, the Charmides, Socrates tells the young Charmides, who has been suffering from headaches, about a charm for headaches that he has recently learnt from one of the mystical physicians to the king of Thrace. According to this physician, however, it is best to cure the soul before curing the body, since health and happiness ultimately depend on the state of the soul.

In recent decades, it has become increasingly clear that psychological stressors can lead to physical symptoms not only by the psychological process of somatization, but also by physical processes involving the nervous, endocrine, and immune systems. For example, one recent study at Harvard Medical School found that the first 24 hours of bereavement are associated with a staggering 21-fold increased risk of a heart attack[1]. Since Robert Ader's initial experiments on laboratory rats in the 1970s, the blossoming field of psychoneuroimmunology has uncovered a large and increasing body of evidence that has led to the mainstream recognition not only of the adverse effects of psychological stress on health, recovery and ageing, but also of the beneficial effects of positive emotions such as happiness, motivation, and a sense of purpose.

The study of psychiatry can do much to broaden and deepen your understanding of health and the good life, even though the poor medical student is seldom given the opportunity to

---

1. Mostofsky E, Maclure M, Sherwood JB et al. (2012), Risk of acute myocardial infarction after the death of a significant person on one's life. The determinants of myocardial infarction onset study. Circulation 2012; 125:491–496.

think beyond the prevalent but reductive and often misguided biological model of mental illness. Tom Bajorek and Tom Stockmann have done a superb job in providing you with all the biological principles that you need to excel in your exams, and have also taken every opportunity to hint and point at some of the richer, more mystical aspects of the specialty, just so that it might not be 2350 years before you rediscover the obvious.

But there are also some more mundane benefits to a career in psychiatry: fascinating patients and plenty of time in which to talk with them, of course, but also broad-minded colleagues, relatively light on calls, and – in most cases – quick career progression. Come on, you'd be a damn fool not to.

Dr Neel Burton
Author of *The Meaning of Madness* and
The Art of Failure
January 2012

Preface

Johann Reil coined the term *psychiatry* in 1808, combining the Ancient Greek words psyche and iatros, meaning *'healing of the soul'*. He thought that psychiatry would be the most challenging branch of medicine, because it involved much more than a physician's or surgeon's knowledge of the body.

Today, psychiatry remains a challenge to many medical students and junior doctors; perceptions of dangerous patients, old-fashioned treatments, and a lack of evidence base, create the illusion of a 'Cinderella' specialty.

With this book, we aim to provide the essential information needed to pass clinical rotations and exams. We also hope that by making the subject accessible, we abolish some of the preconceptions and fears about psychiatry, and inspire further exploration.

We have organised the book as follows: chapters on first principles covering the general topics of patient assessment and management concepts; clinical chapters covering the key disorders, and including example scenarios and practical advice, such as how to approach unwell patients; finally, a chapter covering important legal aspects.

In our opinion, psychiatry is not only the most challenging specialty, but also the most engaging and fascinating. One of the criticisms levelled at psychiatry is the inherent ambiguity. However, it is precisely the unparalleled mix of scientific method, humanity and philosophical exploration that makes psychiatry worthy of pursuit.

Here was the empirical field common to biological and spiritual facts, which I had everywhere sought and nowhere found.
Carl Jung (1875-1961), on choosing psychiatry as a career

Tom Bajorek
Tom Stockmann
January 2012

Contents

Acknowledgements

To AL, PB & RB.
TB

To Natalie, and my parents.
TS

Thank you to Paul Mayhew, Richard Furn and Katrina Rimmer at JP Medical Publishers, for their guidance and patience.
TB, TS

Psychiatric assessment

1.1 Assessment of the patient

Personal safety

Psychiatric patients are usually vulnerable, but a minority can pose a threat to the safety of others. Always keep in mind your personal safety:

- use previous records and colleagues' assessments to gauge the potential risk
- consider a chaperone (out of sight if possible); take care not to 'crowd' the patient
- carry a personal alarm, and be familiar with any alarm system
- choose a suitable room with adequate space and no obstructions or potential weapons
- sit nearest the exit, without blocking the patient's escape route
- be calm and reassuring; avoid rushing, distractions and interrogation, and maintain a relaxed body language
- be alert for signs of agitation, e.g. staring, clenched fists, changes in speech, forward-leaning posture and pacing
- if you do not feel safe, leave calmly and politely

The history

The history is of key importance in psychiatry. This is not only because physical examination and investigations are usually of only limited use, but also because allowing patients to tell their stories, express their fears and anxieties, while being truly listened to and understood (perhaps for the first time), is a powerful therapeutic process.

The history can be divided as follows:
- basic information

- presenting complaint and history of the presenting complaint
- past psychiatric history
- past medical history
- treatment history
- substance use
- family history
- personal history
- social history
- collateral history

Basic information

Before seeing patients, note their age, sex, ethnic/cultural background, occupation, status with respect to relevant mental health legislation, such as the Mental Health Act in England and Wales, and the referral details.

Presenting complaint and history of the presenting complaint

After introducing yourself to the patient, use an open question to allow the patient to start telling their story, such as:
- How are things?
- What's going on?
- What brings you here today?

If the patient has several problems, record them all, and identify the most troubling to that patient. For each symptom, establish its:
- nature (ideally in the patient's own words)
- onset
- course
- severity and effect on the patient's life, and their view of the symptom(s)
- precipitating and perpetuating factors
- treatments so far, and their effect
- previous episodes

While taking the history, look out for clues that point to a diagnosis, and then test your hypothesis with targeted questions. For example, if you suspect that the patient's complaint of being tired all the time is due to depression, ask about other expected symptoms, such as low mood, anhedonia, and psychological and somatic symptoms (see **Chapter 4**).

Past psychiatric history

The patient's past psychiatric history can provide information that can aid diagnosis. Ask about any previous:
- psychiatric disorders: diagnoses, severity, chronology
- psychiatric treatments and their effectiveness, e.g. medication, electroconvulsive therapy, psychology
- psychiatric services used: admissions to psychiatric hospitals (dates, durations, whether informal or compulsory); home treatment team, outpatient treatments, day hospital; others, such as patient groups
- history of self-harm or harm to others

Past medical history

Ask patients about any current and previous medical or surgical conditions.

Treatment history

To determine the patient's treatment history, ask about:
- any current medications: name, dose, side-effects, compliance
- any recent changes in medication
- use of over-the-counter medication/herbal medication, e.g. St John's wort for depression or *Ginkgo biloba* for memory problems
- any other non-prescribed medication used, e.g. from their partner or friend
- any allergies or adverse reactions
- current psychological therapy

Substance use

Patients should be asked whether they use:
- alcohol
- illicit drugs
- tobacco

To elicit additional information, use further questioning as appropriate (see **Chapter 8**).

Family history

It is important to ask about a family history of mental disorder or substance dependency. A family tree may be useful for this.

Personal history

The personal history is the 'story' of the patient's life. Some key areas to cover are listed in **Table 1.1**.

Social history

Aspects to cover in the social history are shown in **Table 1.2**.

Before ending, ask the patient whether there is anything else that they would like to mention.

Collateral history

If feasible, further information should be gathered from others, such as close friends, family or carers. Other sources, depending on the situation, may include the police, school teachers or social workers. Consent must be sought from the patient before taking an informant history.

A collateral history is helpful if the patient cannot provide a full history themselves, because, for example, they:
- have psychomotor retardation
- lack insight
- have cognitive impairment
- are intoxicated

It also allows for assessment of the attitude of others to the patient and their problems, and an opportunity to explain the condition and discuss management.

The mental state examination

The mental state examination (MSE) complements the psychiatric history by providing a snapshot of all the patient's symptoms and signs at that point in time. There is considerable overlap between the history and the MSE. Although usually carried out after the history, the MSE also fits appropriately **within** the history, directly after the history of the presenting complaint.

The MSE is divided into seven sections: 1. appearance and behaviour, 2. speech, 3. mood (plus anxiety and risk assessment), 4. thoughts, 5. perception, 6. cognition, 7. insight

Aspect of personal history	Questions to ask
Childhood	Pregnancy and birth: does the patient know of any problems? Developmental milestones: did the patient reach them by the normal time?
Growing up	Childhood: was it happy? Family: ask the patient to describe the people they grew up with Any emotional problems and support received? Traumatic events, e.g. abuse or serious illnesses
School	Was school enjoyable? Was the patient bullied, or did they bully others? Academic record: ask the patient to describe it Any learning disabilities and support received?
Occupation	Chronological list of jobs, and reasons for changes How does the patient find their current job? Any military service?
Relationships	Sexual orientation Chronological list of relationships and their quality, including sexual aspects Partners: age or age at death, occupation, health Any children from their relationships: age or age at death, schooling/occupation, health? Any personal physical or sexual abuse? What support has the patient received for this?
Forensic history	Has the patient ever had problems with the police? Charges, convictions or periods of imprisonment: ask for details
Religious orientation	How important is religion to the patient?
Premorbid personality	How would the patient describe themselves before they became unwell? How do they imagine others would describe them?

Table 1.1 Personal history

Appearance and behaviour

Table 1.3 shows aspects of appearance and behaviour to note during the MSE.

Aspect of social history	Questions to ask
Family	Support: ask the patient to describe the support they receive from their family and their family's attitude to their problems Situation at home: who is there, how is the atmosphere? Other social support
Friendships	Are there people in whom the patient can confide? What other support does the patient receive, e.g. groups, charities Any negative influences, e.g. people who encourage substance misuse, encourage stigma
Housing	Ask for details of the patient's housing, e.g. owned/rented, state of repair, space, any problems?
Self-care	Does the patient have any problems coping with activities of daily living? Do they receive any support for this?
Finances	Any problems? Do they receive any support for this?
Activities	What does the patient do in a typical day? What are their interests and hobbies?

Table 1.2 Social history

Guiding principle

Performing the mental state examination requires a good knowledge of **descriptive psychopathology** – the symptoms and signs of psychiatric disorders. Simple initial questions are used to screen for all significant symptoms and signs; any positive findings are then explored in detail.

Note that psychomotor agitation/retardation describes an alteration of both motor and mental activity.

Catatonia This is a motor syndrome associated with various conditions, including psychotic disorders and affective disorders. It has become less common since the introduction of antipsychotic medication. Catatonia is present if at least two of the five features described in **Table 1.4** are prominent.

Aspect of appearance/ behaviour	Features	Notes
Level of consciousness	Alert	
	Hyperalert	Seen in mania
	Somnolent	Seen in sleep deprivation
Physical appearance	Ethnicity	
	General condition	Any evidence of self-neglect
	Build	
	Grooming, hygiene	
	Attire	Bright, clashing clothes or nudity in mania
	Bodily stigmata	Scars from self-harm or trauma (e.g. piercings, tattoos, needle marks)
	Poor eye contact Sad facial expression Hunched body	Seen in depression
Behaviour and attitude	Quality of rapport	How does he make you feel?
	Eye contact Facial expression Body language	Poor eye contact, sad expression, hunched posture seen in depression
Level of motor activity	Bradykinesia/motor retardation	Reduced motor activity Seen in schizophrenia and depression
	Stupor	Extreme lack of activity: static, mute, unresponsive to stimuli
Disorders of movement	Extrapyramidal	Side-effects of antipsychotic medication
	Tics	Rapid, involuntary, repetitive, purposeless motor movements or vocalisations (see Chapter 12)
	Motor perseveration	Continued repetition of a requested action after it is no longer appropriate
	Catatonia	See **Table 1.4**

Table 1.3 Examples of appearance and behaviour to note during the mental state examination and possible psychiatric disorders that they may signify

Feature	Description
Motor immobility	Stupor, or Catalepsy (waxy flexibility or flexibilitas cerea): the patient's limbs can be manipulated into any posture, after which they are maintained for an unusually long period of time
Motor excitement	Seemingly purposeless and not driven by external stimuli
Negativism	Seemingly purposeless resistance to instructions or physical attempts to be moved
Posturing or Stereotypies or Mannerisms	The patient adopts and maintains unusual and uncomfortable body postures for long periods of time Unusual, repetitive, non-goal-directed movements, e.g. head banging Unusual, repetitive, goal-directed movement, e.g. pulling up socks
Echolalia or Echopraxia	Senseless, parrot-like imitation of another person's speech The abnormal imitation of the actions of another person

Table 1.4 Catatonia: at least two features should be present

Speech

Assess the amount, rate, volume and tone of the patient's speech, as well as the form of speech, which may be a manifestation of a disorder of the form of thought (**formal thought disorder**). The content of speech reflects the patient's thoughts, and is summarised in **Table 1.5**.

Mood

Current mood Assess the patient's current mood, recording both
- your **objective** assessment, e.g. depressed
- their **subjective** description, e.g. 'awful'

Types of mood and their descriptors are shown in **Table 1.6**.

Affect In addition to recording the patient's mood, their affect should also be recorded. A common phrase is that **affect is**

Aspect and type	Further information
Amount, spontaneity	
Logorrhoea	Increased amount of speech (e.g. mania, anxiety, substance abuse)
Poverty of speech	Decreased amount of speech (e.g. depression, chronic schizophrenia)
Rate	
Pressure of speech	Speech is increased in amount and rate, and may be difficult to interrupt (e.g. mania, anxiety)
Speech retardation	The opposite of pressured speech (e.g. depression, chronic schizophrenia)
Mutism	A lack of speech, for which there is no physical explanation
Volume	
Speech volume	For example, can be reduced in depression, or increased in mania
Tone	
Speech tone	For example, monotonal in depression
Form	
Circumstantiality	Excessive details delay reaching the eventually achieved goal of speech
Tangentiality	Answers proceed at a barely related tangent to the question asked
Clang association	Successive words are linked by sound rather than meaning, this may be the manifestation of flight of ideas (see Thoughts section) in mania
Derailment/Knight's move thinking	Speech switches abruptly from one to another, unrelated topic
Word salad	All association between words is lost. Word salad and derailment may be manifestations of a loosening of associations (see section 3.2)
Echolalia	Senseless, parrot-like imitation of another person's speech
Neologism	The use of a new word
Metonym	The use of an existing word with a new meaning attached

Table 1.5 Assessment of a patient's speech: aim to record verbatim examples where these would be useful

Mood	Descriptor
Euthymic	Normal
Depressed	–
Anxious	–
Irritable	–
Elated	Marked happiness (e.g. normal, hypomania, mania)
Euphoric	Undue, exaggerated happiness (e.g. mania, organic brain lesions)
Ecstatic	A subjective experience of the patient and the Universe being one (e.g. normal, mania, schizophrenia, organic disorders)
Apathetic	An absence of feeling (e.g. schizophrenia)
Perplexed	Bafflement (e.g. schizophrenia)

Table 1.6 Types of mood and their descriptors

to mood as weather is to climate. In other words, affect is an observable behaviour reflecting changing emotions (e.g. joy or sadness); mood is a sustained emotional state (e.g. elation or depression).

The types of affect and their descriptors are shown in **Table 1.7**. If you suspect the presence of a mood disorder, explore this further (see **Chapter 4**).

Risk of harm to self or others Ensure that you ask the patient about thoughts of self-harm and suicide if you have not already done so, e.g. 'Have you ever been so low that you felt that life was no longer worth living?'

If there is the suggestion of risk from self-harm or suicide, explore this further (see **Chapter 5**). It is also crucial to enquire about thoughts of harming others.

Thoughts

Assess the stream, form and content of thought. There are overlaps between stream and form of thought; one type of classification is shown in **Table 1.8**, but this is not fixed.

Affect	Descriptor
Normal	–
Reactive	Normal reactions to the emotional content of the discussion (e.g. smiling when speaking about pleasurable topics)
Expansive	Lacking restraint with emotional expression (e.g. mania)
Constricted	Mildly reduced range and intensity of emotional expression
Blunted/flattening (usually used interchangeably)	Marked reduction/lack of range and intensity of emotional expression (e.g. schizophrenia, depression, organic brain disorders)
Labile	Abrupt, disproportionate shifts in affect (e.g. mania, frontal lobe lesions, intoxication)
Emotional incontinence	Total loss of control over affect (e.g. dementia)
Incongruent	Affect does not correlate with the thought content, e.g. laughter when discussing the death of a spouse (e.g. schizophrenia)

Table 1.7 Descriptors of affect

Perception

Assess the patient for distorted perceptions (**sensory distortions**) and false perceptions (**illusions** and **hallucinations**).

Sensory distortions These include distortions of form, intensity, proportions and colour. Ask the patient: 'Have you noticed any changes in the way you see, hear, smell, or taste things?'

Illusions An illusion is a false perception of a real stimulus, i.e. a misinterpretation of a

Guiding principle

Delusions

The different types of delusions and their descriptors are summarised in **Table 1.9**.

Delusions vs overvalued ideas

- **Delusion:** a fixed belief that is held in the face of evidence to the contrary, not explained by culture or religion. It is usually, but not necessarily, false and the process by which the belief is reached is illogical and outlandish. Examples of delusional themes are shown in **Table 1.10**

- **Overvalued idea:** a single atypical but acceptable belief, firmly held but not fixed (cf. a fixed delusion or subjectively senseless obsession), that dominates the person's life

Characteristic	Type	Description
Stream	Pressure of thought	A high variety of thoughts rapidly arise and pass through the mind, causing pressure of speech (e.g. mania, schizophrenia)
	Retardation (or poverty) of thought	The opposite of pressure of thought, resulting in poverty of speech (e.g. depression, schizophrenia)
	Thought block	A sudden loss of the train of thought. The experience is more profound than the normal experience of the 'mind going blank' in anxiety (e.g. schizophrenia)
	Verbal perseveration	The repetition of the same reply (thought) to different questions (e.g. dementia)
Form	Flight of ideas	Thoughts jump rapidly from one idea to another, with only vague connections, such as clang associations, rhymes or puns (e.g. mania)
	Loosening of associations	Thoughts jump rapidly from one idea to another with no apparent connection. This results in muddled speech (e.g. schizophrenia)
	Overinclusive thinking	A loosening of the usual conceptual boundaries, resulting in circumstantiality (e.g. mania)
	Concrete thinking	An inability to understand abstract concepts; can be demonstrated by literal understanding of proverbs or idioms such as 'in a nutshell' (e.g. schizophrenia)
Content	Preoccupations	
	Ruminations	Repetitive and pointless internal debates
	Obsessions and compulsive acts	See Chapter 7
	Phobias	See Chapter 7
	Delusions and overvalued ideas	Also see Chapter 3

Table 1.8 Classification of thoughts

Type	Descriptor
Primary delusion	A new, fully formed delusional idea arising 'out of the blue', with no origin in existing psychopathology or link to previous ideas and events. It may, however, follow delusional mood, or delusional perception
Delusional mood	A period during which the affected person feels that the world seems somehow different, strange or sinister, but he cannot quite tell why. The sudden emergence of a primary delusion or delusional perception during this time provides a relieving explanation (e.g. a patient suddenly realises that she is Joan of Arc, explaining her recent vague sense of being persecuted)
Delusional perception	A (primary) delusional meaning is given to a normal perception (e.g. 'I saw a red telephone box and immediately knew that the aliens had been behind this plot to incarcerate me')
Secondary delusion	A delusion that is secondary to other psychopathology (e.g. a mood disorder, auditory hallucination, other delusion)
Idea of reference	The feeling that other people, objects or chance events hold a special significance for oneself (e.g. 'It seemed that everyone on the bus was talking about me, but of course they weren't')
Delusion of reference	As per idea of reference, but a fixed belief (e.g. a person with persecutory delusions believes that they received a coded message from a television presenter)
Delusional misinterpretation	A patient gives a new meaning to a percept in order to align it with their pre-existing delusional belief (e.g. a person with persecutory delusions attributes static on a telephone line to MI5 listening in)
Systematised delusions	A group of delusions based around a shared theme, or a number of elaborations of one delusion
Folie à deux	A psychotic person conveys his delusion to another person, producing a shared psychotic disorder.

Table 1.9 Types of delusions and their descriptors

Type of delusion	Theme
Delusions of control	Delusions that the control of one's thoughts, feelings or actions are no longer one's own, e.g. thought insertion, thought withdrawal, thought broadcast, passivity of affect/volition/actions, and somatic passivity (see Chapter 3)
Delusions of persecution	Delusions that one is being persecuted, e.g. being pursued by MI5
Delusions of misidentification	Examples include: Capgras syndrome: the delusion that a familiar individual has been replaced by an identical-looking imposter Fregoli syndrome: the delusion that a familiar individual is disguising themselves as a stranger
Delusions of grandeur	Delusions of being special in some way, e.g. being a world-famous rock star or having invented the cure for HIV. There is an overlap with religious delusions
Religious delusions	Delusions of having a special relationship with God/a supernatural power, e.g. of being the Second Coming of Jesus or of being persecuted by the Devil
Delusions of guilt	Delusions of having committed some great wrongdoing, such as a heinous crime for which one deserves punishment or being personally responsible for a tsunami
Nihilistic delusions	Delusions that one (or sometimes another) no longer exists, or is subject to an imminent catastrophe such as death or the end of the world
Somatic (hypochondriacal) delusions	Delusions about the body, e.g. of having an illness or disfigurement
Delusions of jealousy	Delusions regarding the unfaithfulness of a partner
Delusions of love/ erotomania (de Clérambault syndrome)	Delusions of being loved by someone, usually a person of higher social status and with whom one has little or no contact

Table 1.10 Delusional themes

stimulus. They often occur in healthy people. Types include:

- **Pareidolic illusion**: formed images arise from equivocal stimuli, e.g. seeing a face in a cloud
- **Completion illusion**: inattention leads to perceiving incomplete objects as complete, e.g. FIAT seen as FLAT
- **Affect illusion**: caused by the current emotional state, e.g. a scared person walking down a dark road sees a figure in a hedge

Hallucinations   A **hallucination** is a perception without a stimulus, whereas a **pseudohallucination** is less vivid and perceived to arise from the mind (i.e. the person has insight). They can be distinguished by asking whether a voice is heard from inside a person's head or from outside.

Hallucinations can be visual, olfactory, gustatory or somatic (**Table 1.11**). Further classifications of hallucinations are shown in **Table 1.12**.

Hypnogogic and **hypnopompic** hallucinations occur around sleep: a hypnogogic hallucination occurs when going to sleep, whereas a hypnopompic hallucination occurs on waking up. They can be:

- visual, auditory or tactile in nature
- normal; they can also occur in a variety of disorders, including delirium, schizophrenia and narcolepsy

Cognition

A brief test of cognition may involve the following:

- **orientation:** to time, place and person (themselves)
- **attention and concentration**, e.g. serial sevens (subtract 7 from 100, and keep going several times)
- **memory:**
  - short term, e.g. recall of a name and address/three objects after a few minutes
  - long term: recent events (e.g. yesterday's breakfast) and more distant (e.g. dates of the Second World War)

If there appears to be impairment of cognition, a more comprehensive assessment should be performed. This is usually the

Modality/types	Characteristics	Associated disorders
Auditory hallucinations	See **Chapter 3**	
Visual hallucinations		Organic illness; uncommon in primary psychiatric conditions
Lilliputian hallucinations	Images of small animals or people, etc.	Delirium tremens
Charles Bonnet syndrome	Simple or complex hallucinations	Significant loss of vision
Autoscopic hallucinations	Images of oneself, seen by the person while 'remaining' in their own body (cf. 'out-of-body' experience)	
Olfactory (smell) hallucinations	Not common, usually unpleasant, e.g. burning rubber	Organic conditions (e.g. temporal lobe epilepsy) and psychiatric conditions
Gustatory (taste) hallucinations	Not common, usually unpleasant, e.g. bitter	Organic conditions (e.g. temporal lobe epilepsy) and psychiatric conditions
Somatic hallucinations	Bodily sensations, e.g. touch/haptic, pain, proprioception, temperature	Schizophrenia (may be incorporated into a complex delusion (e.g. the sensation of being touched lends further evidence to persecution by another person)
Formication	Haptic hallucination of insects crawling on or under the skin (e.g. 'cocaine bugs' in cocaine intoxication)	Alcohol withdrawal, cocaine addiction

Table 1.11 Hallucinatory modalities

'gold standard' 30-point Folstein **mini-mental state examination** (MMSE), which provides an assessment of:
- orientation
- registration (immediate memory)

Type	Examples
Simple (or elementary) hallucinations	Simple sounds such as a bang, or simple flashes of light
Complex hallucinations	Complex sounds such as music/voices, or complex images of objects/people
Functional hallucinations	Hallucinations triggered by a simultaneous external stimulus of the *same* modality, e.g. hallucinatory voices heard when the toilet is heard flushing
Reflex hallucinations	Hallucinations triggered by a simultaneous external stimulus in a *different* modality, e.g. a visual hallucination seen when a door is heard creaking
Synaesthesia (non-hallucinatory form of reflex hallucinations)	Stimuli in one modality leads to sensations in another, e.g. experiencing a song as a stream of colours. Can occur in the absence of illness
Extracampine hallucinations	Hallucinations perceived as from outside the limits of the sensory field, e.g. hearing astronauts speaking on the moon

Table 1.12 Further classification of hallucinations

- short-term memory
- language

The UK National Institute for Health and Clinical Excellence (NICE) classifies the degree of cognitive impairment according to the MMSE score as follows:

25–30	normal
21–24	mild
10–20	moderate
<10	severe

Insight

Insight is the degree of understanding that a person has of their illness and its impact. It exists on a spectrum, rather than just being present or not.

Clinical insight

The mini-mental state examination may produce false-positive results in various cultural groups and those with low education or intelligence. Conversely, it may not reveal subtle cognitive impairment, especially in intelligent or well-educated patients.

'Poor insight' is characteristic of certain mental disorders, including mania, schizophrenia and dementia.

Determine whether the patient believes that they are unwell by asking, for example:

- Do you think there is anything wrong with you?
- Why did you come to hospital?

If the patient does feel that they are unwell, assess their understanding or belief of what their illness is:

- What do you think is wrong with you?
- What do you think the cause of it is?
- Do you think you need treatment?
- What are you hoping treatment will do for you?
- Do you think you need to come into hospital?

1.2 Formulation

The formulation is a clinical opinion. It reviews the most important points ascertained from the history and examination and weighs up the evidence for and against possible diagnoses before discussion of management and prognosis, according to:

- case synopsis
- further information required
- differential diagnosis
- aetiology
- management plan including risk assessment
- prognosis

Case synopsis

This should include:

- background information (including the patient's name, age, occupation)
- presenting complaint
- a summary of the main findings

Further information required

This may include further patient interview, collateral history, access to old notes, physical examination, laboratory investigations, imaging, psychological testing and inpatient observation.

Differential diagnoses
It is important to start this process with the most probable diagnosis first and the least likely diagnosis last. For each proposed diagnosis, factors for and against should be presented. Points to bear in mind include the diagnostic hierarchy (**Figure 1.1**) and the possibility of comorbid (dual) diagnoses.

Aetiology
From the history, outline the predisposing, precipitating and maintaining factors in the patient's presentation, as well as the protective factors. These can be subclassified using the **biopsychosocial model** as biological, psychological or social. It may be useful to create a table of aetiological factors and then consider which may be removed, modified or reversed as part of the management plan (**Table 1.13**).

Management plan
A holistic plan (i.e. one including psychological and social dimensions not just biological ones) is critical since medication on its own will solve few problems. It may be useful to divide the management plan into short-, medium- and long-term interventions (**Table 1.14**). The plan should also detail who is responsible for each aspect of care, what the timescale for implementation is and when the problem will be reviewed.

Risk assessment
All patients should have a risk assessment considering a broad range of risks (**Table 1.15**). When assessing risk:
- review former notes in addition to the current situation and mental state, as past behaviour is the best predictor of future behaviour
- review regularly as risk is sensitive to changing circumstances
- each domain identified as a risk should have an estimate of likelihood, seriousness and immediacy, and the factors affecting it

	Biological	Psychological	Social
Predisposing factors	Genetic factors Family history Substance abuse Organic conditions	Cognitive distortions Maladaptive behaviours (e.g. impulsive/violent) Psychodynamic factors Poor parenting	Childhood abuse Bullying Lack of social support Accommodation issues Unemployment
Precipitating factors	Organic conditions Substance abuse Non-compliance with medication Sleep pattern	Bereavement Stress (real or perceived)	Life events
Maintaining factors	Organic conditions Substance abuse Non-compliance Treatment resistance Sleep pattern	Poor insight Personality traits High expressed emotion Paucity of confiding relationships Maladaptive behaviours	Stigma Poor social support Poor housing Unemployment
Protective factors	No family history of mental illness No substance misuse Responsive to medication Compliance with medication	Good insight Motivated to recover Confiding relationships	Good premorbid function Good social support Employment

Table 1.13 The biopsychosocial model of common aetiological factors

- balance risk reduction (e.g. through detention under mental health legislation) with the human rights of the individual

Prognosis

Describe a clear prognosis for both the current episode and the longer term, explaining your rationale. A list of relevant positive and negative prognostic factors may be useful (**Table 1.13**).

	Short term	Medium and long term
Biological	Medication Electroconvulsive therapy Detoxification Treatment of comorbid medical conditions	Regular review Maintenance treatment Depot antipsychotic Mood stabiliser Treatment of addiction
Psychological	Counselling Psychoeducation	Bibliotherapy Psychological therapies such as problem-solving therapy, cognitive–behavioural therapy, family therapy
Social	Family education Carer support Carer respite	Patient groups (weight loss, self-esteem, etc.) Charities Benefits Housing Employment Power of attorney

Table 1.14 Possible interventions for mental disorders according to the biopsychosocial model

1.3 Classification of psychiatric disorders

After assessing a patient's problems there are two main ways of thinking about mental illness. The first is the **ideographic approach**, which avoids classifying abnormal behaviour into diagnostic groupings; instead, each patient is analysed individually. The second approach is the **nomothetic approach**, which classifies and categorises disorders. This is the prevailing way in which psychiatric services approach mental illness.

Difficulties with classification in psychiatry
Syndromes not diseases
Many psychiatric diagnoses are syndromes i.e. a constellation of symptoms rather than distinct diseases with a clear aetiology.

Factor	Examples
Harm to self	Attempted suicide Suicidal ideation Self-harm Self-neglect
Harm to others	Violence or aggression/abuse of family Violence or aggression/abuse of other service users Violence or aggression to staff Violence or aggression to the general public Hostage-taking Possession of weapons Sexual assault Arson Stalking Emotional or financial exploitation Neglect of children or dependents
Harm from others	Physical harm Sexual exploitation Emotional or psychological abuse Financial abuse Withholding of personal rights, e.g. locking doors/ withholding food/treatment
Other risks	Arrest/detention by police Damage to property Inappropriate phone calls, especially to emergency services Non-compliance with medication or treatment plan Absconding Wandering Accidents Falls Unsafe use of medication Driving/road safety
Factors affecting risk	Current mental state: anger; delusions of persecution, control or guilt; command hallucinations; lack of insight Nature of illness: depression, psychosis, treatment difficulties Recent life events/stressors Access to means Substance misuse Non-compliance with medication Housing status Lack of insight Nature of condition Provision of support/resources available to contain the patient

Table 1.15 Risk assessment

Unlike other medical specialties, there is usually no laboratory or radiological 'proof' for psychiatric diagnoses. Unsurprisingly the validity of almost all disorders has come to be questioned at some point.

Loss of individuality/dual diagnosis/causation

One criticism of psychiatric classification systems is that they pigeonhole individuals and apply diagnostic labels to them. Also, many patients may have more than one psychiatric disorder. It is well established that having one psychiatric disorder increases the risk of having another and that over 50% of psychiatric patients have two or more diagnoses. Furthermore, two disorders may or may not be causally related, e.g. a patient with known cardiovascular disease and vascular dementia compared with a patient with lifelong bipolar disorder and breast cancer. The multiaxial systems go some way to resolving these problems.

Disorder 'importance'

There is a tradition of hierarchical diagnosis in psychiatry. Therefore, when an organic disorder such as a brain tumour is present, coexisting disorders tend not to be diagnosed. Similarly, psychotic illness traditionally 'trumps' neurosis because of the belief that, if the 'higher' problem is treated, the 'lower' one will disappear. Unfortunately, in practice, this is not always the case. **Figure 1.1** shows the hierarchy of diagnoses.

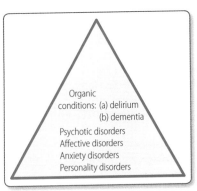

Figure 1.1 The diagnostic hierarchy of psychiatric disorders.

Classification systems

Despite these problems, categorical diagnosis are important in gaining an understanding of the patient, communicating information with colleagues and providing rational treatment and prognostication. It is also critical in facilitating good research.

There are two main classification systems, both of which are categorical: the ICD-10 and DSM-IV. In reality, both systems are broadly similar and are used to varying extents by different practitioners.

ICD-10

The 10th revision of the International Classification of Diseases (ICD-10) is a classificatory system intended for all medical disorders that is produced by the World Health Organization. It consists of 21 chapters, with psychiatric disorders described in Chapter V. As well as listing and coding diseases and disorders, it provides clinical descriptions and diagnostic criteria. These are based on available scientific evidence, consultation and expert consensus.

Diagnoses are preceded by the letter F and are listed in a broadly hierarchical fashion:

F00–F09 Organic, including symptomatic, mental disorders
F10–F19 Mental and behavioural disturbances due to psychoactive substance use
F20–F29 Schizophrenia, schizotypal and delusional disorders
F30–F39 Mood (affective) disorders
F40–F48 Neurotic, stress-related and somatoform disorders
F50–F59 Behavioural syndromes associated with physiological disturbances and physical factors
F60–F69 Disorders of adult personality and behaviour
F70–F79 Mental retardation
F80–F90 Disorders of psychological development
F90–F98 Behavioural and emotional disorders with onset usually occurring in childhood and adolescence

There are four different versions of ICD-10:
1. clinical descriptions and diagnostic guidelines
2. diagnostic criteria for research

Axis	Classification
I	Clinical disorders and the conditions that need clinical attention
II	Personality disorders and mental retardation
III	General medical conditions
IV	Psychosocial and environmental problems
V	Global assessment of functioning

Table 1.16 Axes of classification in DSM-IV

3. a primary care version
4. a multiaxial version

DSM-IV

The Diagnostic and Statistical Manual of Mental Disorders, which is currently in its fourth revision (DSM-IV), is an alternative classificatory system published by the American Psychiatric Association. It describes only mental disorders and is a multiaxial system with set operational criteria. This means that, for a diagnosis to be made, a given number of symptoms need to have been present for a given duration. The five axes are given in **Table 1.16**.

Management

2.1 Antidepressants

Table 2.1 shows the different antidepressant classes.

Tricyclic antidepressants

TCAs inhibit the reuptake of noradrenaline and serotonin, as well as acting as antagonists at various other receptors (**Table 2.2**). A higher rate of side-effects and greater toxicity in overdose means that they are used less frequently than selective serotonin reuptake inhibitors (SSRIs), and they should be used with particular caution in the elderly and physically ill.

Selective serotonin reuptake inhibitors

SSRIs inhibit the reuptake of serotonin by presynaptic neurones, increasing the amount of serotonin in the synaptic cleft available to bind with postsynaptic receptors. The side-effects of SSRI use are shown in **Table 2.3**.

Monoamine oxidase inhibitors

Monoamine oxidase inhibitors (MAOIs) reduce the breakdown of monoamine neurotransmitters by monoamine oxidase. With the exception of moclobemide, MAOIs are now rarely prescribed, because of the risk of the potentially fatal **tyramine reaction** (the 'cheese and chianti' reaction). This is a hypertensive crisis caused by interaction between the medication and foods rich in tyramine, such as cheese, game, yeast extracts and sympathomimetic drugs (e.g. some cold remedies). The side-effects of MAOIs include:

- postural hypotension
- dizziness
- sleep disturbances
- oedema
- paraesthesiae
- anticholinergic effects

Type of antidepressant	Examples
Monoamine oxidase inhibitor (MAOI) Non-specific	Phenelzine
Reversible inhibitor of monoamine oxidase A (RIMA)	Tranylcypromine
	Moclobemide
Tricyclic antidepressant (TCA)	Amitriptyline
	Imipramine
Selective serotonin reuptake inhibitor (SSRI)	Citalopram
	Escitalopram
	Sertraline
	Fluoxetine
	Paroxetine
Serotonin–noradrenaline reuptake inhibitor (SNRI)	Venlafaxine
	Duloxetine
Noradrenaline reuptake inhibitor (NRI)	Reboxetine
Noradrenaline and specific serotonin antidepressant (NaSSA)	Mirtazapine
Serotonin agonist and reuptake inhibitor (SARI)	Trazodone
Melatonergic agonist and serotonin antagonist	Agomelatine

Table 2.1 Antidepressant classifications

Type	Side-effect
Cardiovascular	Arrhythmias, ECG changes (e.g. prolonged QT interval, T wave changes)
Neurological	Seizures, delirium
Anticholinergic	Dry mouth, blurred vision, raised intraocular pressure, constipation, urinary retention
Serotonin blockade	Sexual dysfunction, weight gain
Antihistaminergic	Sedation, weight gain
α-Adrenoceptor blockade	Postural hypotension

Table 2.2 Side-effects of tricyclic antidepressants

Side-effect	Example/notes
Gastrointestinal upset	Nausea/vomiting, diarrhoea, abdominal pain, anorexia
Hypersensitivity reactions	Rash
Sexual dysfunction	Erectile dysfunction, anorgasmia
Insomnia	–
Headache, dizziness	–
Anxiety, sweating, restlessness	–
Dry mouth	–
Hyponatraemia	Particularly significant in the elderly
Increased bleeding tendency	–
Tremor, dystonia	–

Table 2.3 Side-effects of selective serotonin reuptake inhibitors

Moclobemide is a reversible inhibitor of monoamine oxidase A. It leaves MAO-B free to metabolise tyramine, rendering dietary and other restrictions unnecessary.

Other antidepressants

Information on other antidepressants is summarised in **Table 2.4**.

Antidepressants in pregnancy and breastfeeding

The risks and key points of the use of antidepressants in pregnancy and breastfeeding are shown in **Table 2.5**.

2.2 Antipsychotics

Typical or first-generation antipsychotics

The first antipsychotics were initially thought to treat psychosis through neurological suppression, as neuroleptics (Greek: *seizing the nerves*). Their clinical potency was later found to correlate with blockade of **dopamine D$_2$** receptors, a finding that contributed to the dopamine theory of schizophrenia (**Chapter 3**).

Antidepressant	Effects
Mirtazapine	Common side-effects include increased appetite and sedation (which can be useful) Relatively low rate of sexual side-effects
Venlafaxine	Side-effect profile similar to that of selective serotonin reuptake inhibitors, plus hypertension ECG and blood pressure monitoring recommended Caution in people with cardiovascular conditions
Trazodone	Related to tricyclic antidepressants, with similar side-effects Particularly sedating In rare cases, causes priapism
Agomelatine	A relatively recent (and expensive) antidepressant with a novel mode of action Promising results in clinical trials but is not currently widely used Thought to have relatively few side-effects, including dizziness and deranged liver function tests

Table 2.4 Summary of the effects of other antidepressants

This D_2 blockade affects dopaminergic pathways other than those involved in psychosis, in particular those involved in motor control, leading to significant **extrapyramidal side-effects** (Table 2.6).

Typical antipsychotics (e.g. chlorpromazine, haloperidol) act on various other receptors (e.g. cholinergic, histaminergic, adrenergic), with corresponding further side-effects (shared with TCAs - see **Table 2.2**).

Atypical or second-generation antipsychotics

Another early drug, clozapine, was also an effective antipsychotic but had a different mode of action, blocking **5-HT$_2$** (5-hydroxytryptamine; serotonin) receptors as well as D_2 receptors. It also had a lower rate of extrapyramidal side-effects, and became known as the first atypical or second-generation antipsychotic.

Clozapine inspired the production of other antipsychotics that also acted on both D_2 and 5-HT$_2$ receptors, which were

Risks	
Antidepressant	Effect
All	Neonatal withdrawal (usually mild and self-limiting)
Selective serotonin reuptake inhibitor (SSRIs)	Persistent neonatal pulmonary hypertension if taken after 20 weeks of pregnancy
Paroxetine	Fetal heart defects if taken in the first trimester
High-dose venlafaxine	Hypertension
Key points	
Antidepressant	Notes
Tricyclic antidepressants (TCAs)	Have the lowest known risks in pregnancy
Fluoxetine	The only SSRI licensed for use in pregnancy

Table 2.5 Antidepressants in pregnancy and breastfeeding

promoted as having greater effectiveness and fewer side-effects than typical antipsychotics.

Atypical antipsychotics (e.g. olanzapine, quetiapine, amisulpride, aripiprazole, risperidone) have complex actions, interacting with many other receptors (e.g. D_1, D_3, D_4; various 5-HT subtypes; cholinergic; histaminergic; adrenergic).

Atypical antipsychotics do tend to have a lower incidence of extrapyramidal symptoms than typical antipsychotics, but have significant side-effects of their own, including increasing the risk of **metabolic syndrome** (obesity, deranged lipids, hypertension, impaired glucose tolerance).

Depot antipsychotics

Some antipsychotics are available in longer acting, injectable forms, known as depot preparations:

- these provide a slow release of the medication over the period between injections (usually two to four weeks)

Side-effect (percentage of patients)	Further information
Dystonia (10%)	Acute or chronic spasms of muscle groups, particularly in younger patients. Oculogyric crises affect the eyes; torticollis involves the head and neck. They may be painful, and are treated with anticholinergics, such as procyclidine or orphenadrine
Parkinsonian-like or pseudo-Parkinsonism (20%)	A triad of resting tremor, bradykinesia and muscle rigidity that can particularly effect the elderly. Management strategies include dose reduction, anticholinergics, or switching to another antipsychotic
Akathisia (25%)	A distressing feeling of inner restlessness and resultant uncontrolled movements such as leg fidgeting. Management involves dose reduction or switching to an atypical antipsychotic; propranolol can also be useful in some cases (but not anticholinergics)
Tardive dyskinesia	Repetitive, involuntary movements that lack purpose, such as lip smacking. It can arise after months or years of antipsychotic use, but is also seen in untreated schizophrenia and even in the healthy elderly. Reductions in dosage, or switching to clozapine or another atypical antipsychotic may be carried out, but tardive dyskinesia is reversible in only 50% of cases

Table 2.6 Extrapyramidal side-effects of antipsychotics

- most are typical antipsychotics, such as haloperidol decanoate and pipotiazine palmitate
- Risperidone was the only atypical available as a depot until the recent introductions of olanzapine and paliperidone (a metabolite of risperidone)

The advantages and disadvantages of depot antipsychotics are shown in **Table 2.7.**

Side-effects of antipsychotics
Extrapyramidal
Extrapyramidal side-effects are shown in **Table 2.6.**

Advantages	Disadvantages
Possibly reduced rate of relapse	Potential harm to the therapeutic relationship
Improved adherence, e.g. easier monitoring, no need to remember a daily tablet	Inflexibility
Regular contact with services (community psychiatric nurse/depot clinic)	Cannot be withdrawn if side-effects occur (test doses used)
Longer therapeutic action	Local side-effects of inflammation (and, less likely, infection) at injection site
Greater consistency of delivery; avoidance of first-pass metabolism	Delayed action
Allows compulsory treatment to be given when patient refuses tablets	–
Less potential for overdose	–

Table 2.7 Advantages and disadvantages of depot antipsychotics

Neuroleptic malignant syndrome

Neuroleptic malignant syndrome (NMS) is a very rare but potentially fatal complication of antipsychotic use.

Overactivation of the sympathetic nervous system may cause:

- autonomic instability
- muscle rigidity and raised creatine kinase (potentially leading to renal failure)
- hyperthermia
- confusion
- elevated leucocytes
- deranged liver function tests (LFTs)

Guiding principle

The typical/atypical classification of antipsychotics is now considered unhelpful:

- There are no significant differences in clinical effectiveness (in everyday practice) between any antipsychotic, apart from clozapine for schizophrenia resistant to other antipsychotics
- Earlier favourable results for atypical efficacy (in trials) were perhaps due to comparing them with (poorly tolerated) high-dose haloperidol
- Each antipsychotic has a signature pattern of receptor action, with a corresponding side-effect profile and efficacy. Differences between individual drugs are perhaps more significant than those between classes

NMS is a medical emergency. Treatment involves stopping the antipsychotic and introducing supportive measures, which may be supplemented by the use of benzodiazepines, dantrolene or bromocriptine.

Other

Other side-effects of antipsychotic drugs are shown in **Table 2.8**. Antipsychotic drug use can lead to **hyperprolactinaemia** by reducing dopaminergic inhibition of prolactin production by the anterior pituitary, possibly causing:

- galactorrhoea
- reduced libido
- erectile dysfunction
- reduced bone density
- amenorrhoea
- gynaecomastia

Antipsychotics in pregnancy and breastfeeding

The risks of antipsychotic drug use in pregnancy and breast-feeding are shown in **Table 2.9**.

2.3 Mood stabilisers

Lithium

Lithium is used for the treatment of mania and the long-term prophylaxis of both bipolar disorder and (less commonly) unipolar depression. It is less effective for the treatment of depression in bipolar disorder, but is sometimes used together with an antidepressant drug for this purpose. Side-effects are shown in **Table 2.10**.

Plasma-level monitoring

There is a narrow window of therapeutic levels of lithium in the blood: 0.4–1.0 mmol/L (although this can vary between laboratories). Levels above this range, and particularly above 1.5 mmol/L, can lead to toxicity.

Patients prescribed lithium must have their plasma levels monitored:

Side-effect	More likely with	Less likely with
Sedation	Chlorpromazine, clozapine	Aripiprazole, sulpiride and amisulpride
Weight gain	Atypical antipsychotics (especially clozapine and olanzapine), although common with all	Aripiprazole
Impaired glucose tolerance: can lead to diabetes	Clozapine, olanzapine, risperidone and quetiapine	Aripiprazole
Dyslipidaemia	Chlorpromazine, clozapine, olanzapine, risperidone and quetiapine	Aripiprazole
Anticholinergic effects	Chlorpromazine and clozapine	Amisulpride
Hyperprolactinaemia	Risperidone and amisulpride	Not caused by clozapine, quetiapine and aripiprazole Transient change only with olanzapine
Hypertension	Clozapine	–
Postural hypotension	Chlorpromazine, clozapine, risperidone and quetiapine	–
QT interval prolongation: increases the risk of torsades de pointes, a potentially fatal cardiac arrhythmia	Haloperidol	Aripiprazole
Reduced seizure threshold	Clozapine	

Table 2.8 Other side-effects of antipsychotics

- One week after the initial dose, and one week after dose change
- weekly until levels are stable

Drug	Risks
Olanzapine	Weight gain and gestational diabetes
Clozapine	Agranulocytosis in the fetus or breastfed baby
	Avoid routine use of clozapine during pregnancy or breastfeeding
All, but especially depots	Extrapyramidal symptoms in the neonate
All but especially risperidone, amisulpride and sulpiride	Increase in prolactin can reduce fertility

Table 2.9 The risks of antipsychotic drug use in pregnancy and breastfeeding

Acute	Chronic
Nausea and diarrhoea	Hypothyroidism, goitre (more rarely, hyperthyroidism)
Dizziness	Hyperparathyroidism
Muscle weakness	Weight gain
Fine tremor	Oedema
Polyuria, polydipsia	Nephrotoxicity, nephrogenic diabetes insipidus
Metallic taste	Cardiotoxicity

Table 2.10 Side-effects of lithium

- every three months thereafter
- anytime if there are signs of lithium toxicity (they can occur at normal levels, however)

Lithium levels are taken 12 hours post dose. Baseline full blood count (FBC), urea and electrolytes (U&Es), thyroid-stimulating hormone (TSH) and weight/body mass index (BMI) must also be taken, with U&Es and TSH monitored 6 monthly. A baseline ECG is recommended, especially with existing cardiovascular disease.

Toxicity

The risk of lithium toxicity is increased by comorbid conditions such as heart failure, hypertension and chronic renal failure.

Signs and symptoms The signs and symptoms of **lithium toxicity** include:
- worsening gastrointestinal upset: diarrhoea, vomiting, anorexia
- coarse tremor, ataxia, reduced co-ordination, dysarthria, muscle weakness
- lethargy, drowsiness, confusion

The signs and symptoms of severe lithium toxicity (usually with lithium levels above 2 mmol/L) include:
- seizures
- dehydration, renal failure, electrolyte disturbances
- cardiovascular collapse, coma, death

Treatment of toxicity involves stopping the lithium and employing supportive measures.

Lithium in pregnancy and breastfeeding

Lithium use in early pregnancy increases the risk of fetal heart defects, e.g. Ebstein's anomaly (abnormalities of the tricuspid valve). Avoid routine use:
- if pregnancy planned
- during pregnancy (particularly in the first trimester)
- during breastfeeding (high levels in breast milk).

Valproate

Valproate semisodium is licensed for the treatment of manic episodes in bipolar disorder. It does not require routine plasma-level monitoring, but baseline FBC, LFTs and BMI should be recorded, with FBC and LFTs repeated six months after initiation.

The side-effects of valproate use include:
- gastrointestinal upset (e.g. nausea)
- weight gain
- lethargy, confusion
- hair loss
- pancreatitis
- blood dyscrasias (e.g. thrombocytopenia and leucopenia)
- liver failure (rare)

Valproate in pregnancy and breastfeeding

The risks include neural tube defects and effects on cognitive development. Avoid routine use in women of child-bearing potential because of the risks to pregnancy. Valproate may be used if there is no alternative, with informed consent and advice on adequate contraception.

Carbamazepine

The anticonvulsant carbamazepine is licensed for the prophylaxis of bipolar disorder if a combination of other mood stabilisers have been ineffective. It is also used for rapid-cycling bipolar disorder (see **Chapter 4**).

Baseline FBC, LFTs and U&Es should be taken, and then monitored, along with carbamazepine plasma levels, every six months.

The side-effects of carbamazepine use include:

- gastrointestinal upset (e.g. nausea and vomiting)
- sedation
- dizziness
- ataxia
- skin reactions (including Stevens–Johnson syndrome)
- hyponatraemia (usually mild)
- blood disorders (e.g. leucopenia, thrombocytopenia, agranulocytosis)
- liver dysfunction or failure
- liver enzyme induction can affect other medication (e.g. the oral contraceptive pill)

Carbamazepine in pregnancy and breastfeeding

Risks include fetal neural tube defects, gastrointestinal upset and cardiac abnormalities. Avoid routine use if pregnancy is planned, or during pregnancy.

Lamotrigine

Lamotrigine is used for the prevention of depressive episodes associated with bipolar disorder. It does not require monitoring of plasma levels.

The side-effects of lamotrigine use include:

- tiredness
- gastrointestinal disturbance (e.g. nausea and vomiting)

- headache
- dizziness
- blurred vision, diplopia
- drowsiness, confusion
- skin rash (rarely Stevens–Johnson syndrome), lupus-like reactions
- blood dyscrasias (e.g. leucopenia, thrombocytopenia)

Lamotrigine in pregnancy and breastfeeding

Risks include:
- oral cleft defects in pregnancy
- dermatological problems (including Stevens–Johnson syndrome) with breastfeeding

Avoid routine use if pregnancy planned, during pregnancy or during breastfeeding.

Benzodiazepines

Chlordiazepoxide, the first benzodiazepine, was discovered serendipitously in the 1950s.

Benzodiazepines act at the benzodiazepine binding site on the inhibitory γ-amino-butyric acid (GABA)-A receptors. They have a range of uses, including:
- treatment of severe anxiety
- treatment of epilepsy
- alleviating symptoms of alcohol withdrawal/detoxification
- treatment of insomnia
- treatment of muscle spasticity
- sedation before operations
- sedation in severe agitation/behavioural disturbance

The half-lives and potencies of benzodiazepines vary, affecting their uses (**Table 2.11**).

Side-effects of benzodiazepines

Limiting the prescription of benzodiazepines to short courses is recommended, as they are associated with dependence and are a drug of abuse.

Abrupt cessation once tolerance has developed may cause withdrawal symptoms, including confusion, psychosis, seizures and delirium tremens (see **Chapter 8**).

Half life	Potency	Drug	Example of use
Short	High	Lorazepam	Rapid sedation
Short	Low	Temazepam	Short-term preoperative sedation
Long	High	Clonazepam	Longer term sedation, anticonvulsant
Long	Low	Chlordiazepoxide	Alcohol detoxification

Table 2.11 Examples of benzodiazepines and their uses according to half-life and potency

Other side-effects include:
- amnesia
- confusion
- ataxia
- muscle weakness
- paradoxical increase in agitation and aggression

Benzodiazepines in pregnancy and breastfeeding
Risks include cleft palate and other fetal malformations and 'floppy baby syndrome'. Avoid routine use in pregnancy (unless required for the short-term management of extreme anxiety and agitation).

2.4 Psychological therapies

Psychological, or 'talking', therapies are effective for a range of psychiatric conditions. In some cases, they may be the preferred intervention; in others, they may be used alongside pharmacological treatment. They may be preferred to medication by those patients who are seeking help with underlying problems, rather than the concealment of surface symptoms.

Supportive psychotherapy
Offering an explanation, support and reassurance is a basic intervention that is important for all patients.

Counselling

This is a short-term treatment, similar to supportive psycho-therapy but focused on helping the patient deal with particular problems.

Cognitive–behavioural therapy

Cognitive–behavioural therapy (CBT) is an evidence-based and cost-effective treatment, developed by Aaron Beck in the 1960s.

In CBT, patients are helped to understand their problems in terms of their cognitions/thoughts, emotional feelings, physical feelings and behaviour, and the links between these.

Goals are then set, using both:

- cognitive techniques, e.g. examining, testing and altering automatic negative beliefs in depression (**thinking errors**), and
- behavioural techniques, e.g. monitoring achievements, scheduling activities, graded exposure to feared situations

These goals are designed to be realistic and time limited, with much of the work taking place outside the sessions (homework).

CBT is usually an individual therapy, although it can be group based. It is usually limited to 8–20 sessions.

Interpersonal therapy

Rather than looking at patients' internal mental processes, interpersonal therapy focuses on identifying and resolving issues in their current personal relationships that are linked to their illness.

Family therapy and couples therapy

Family therapy and couples therapy assist those involved to discover and resolve problems in their relationships that are contributing to their mental disorder.

Psychodynamic psychotherapy

The aim of psychodynamic psychotherapy is to assist the person to identify and understand unconscious feelings from their past that affect their present thoughts, emotions and behaviour, and thus contribute to their mental health issues.

2.5 Electroconvulsive therapy

Electroconvulsive therapy (ECT) involves using electrical stimulation of the brain to induce a convulsion. It is only recommended for rapid and short-term improvement of severe symptoms unresponsive to all other treatment options, or as a life-saving measure, in:

- a severe depressive illness
- a prolonged or severe episode of mania
- catatonia

It remains unknown how ECT actually works, although hypotheses include an increase in neurotransmitters (such as serotonin) or increased numbers or sensitivity of their receptors, as well as stimulation of cerebral blood vessel growth.

> ### Guiding principle
>
> Electroconvulsive therapy (ECT) can be given only under two conditions:
>
> - when a patient has capacity (see **Chapter 13**) and gives informed consent or
> - when a patient does not have capacity to give or refuse consent but ECT is deemed 'appropriate' and does not conflict with a valid advance decision, or a decision made by a donee, deputy or by the relevant court (in England and Wales, for example, this is the Court of Protection)
>
> In the UK, the Mental Health Act 2007 prohibits ECT use in a patient who is judged to have capacity and refuses treatment.

Method

A general anaesthetic and muscle relaxant is administered before electrodes are placed on the patient's temples and a current passed through the brain. The induced generalised seizure is monitored using an electroencephalograph (EEG) recording.

Patients usually have 6–12 sessions of ECT, usually with two sessions per week. The side-effects of ECT are shown in **Table 2.12.**

Short-term	Long-term
Transient recent memory loss	Memory problems
Headache	Long-term anterograde and
Nausea	retrograde memory loss
Muscle ache	
Cardiovascular effects	
General anaesthetic risks: including	
a 1 in 50,000 risk of death or serious	
injury	

Table 2.12 Side-effects of electroconvulsive therapy

Clinical insight

As electroconvulsive therapy (ECT) can be life-saving, there are no absolute contraindications. Relative contraindications include the following (note not age or pregnancy):

- recent stroke or myocardial infarction
- raised intracranial pressure
- severe cardiac failure
- unstable major fracture

Schizophrenia

3.1 Clinical scenario

A patient 'behaving strangely'

Presentation

27-year-old Anna was brought in to the emergency department by the police (under the relevant mental health legislation - see **Chapter 13**). She is now in the medical assessment ward.

The police, alerted by an intruder alarm, found her wandering around a church in the early hours. She was in wet clothes on a chilly evening. She did not respond when approached, and appeared to be bleeding from both palms. They found her personal details in her belongings and visited her address, which was in a poor state of repair and uninhabitable.

Anna expressed persecutory ideas to emergency department staff, such as 'The Devil is inside me', and spoke of being bitten by vampires. She feared that the doctors were going to bite her, and did not co-operate with a physical examination. They were only able to clean and inspect her wounds, which were superficial, and to take routine blood tests, which were unremarkable. She later received lorazepam because of aggression towards staff.

Diagnostic approach

Her symptoms indicate psychosis, and that she is at risk of harm to herself. She has had blood tests, but will require the completion of her physical examination when possible and a drug test to rule out common 'organic' causes of psychosis.

She requires a full psychiatric review and risk assessment.

Initial history

In the initial interview, she does not answer any questions directly. She appears perplexed and preoccupied, constantly looking around the room. She states fearfully that 'He … the

Devil ... wants me dead', and repeatedly that 'I can feel my soul being taken from my body'.

Her facial expressions do not reflect her speech, which itself is sometimes difficult to comprehend, as her thoughts seem disjointed.

She frequently gets up and wanders over to the window, where she alternately holds out her arms or appears to pray, while saying that 'the Holy Spirit is in the sky … it wants to go inside me …'.

Diagnostic approach

It was not possible to establish a full history, but the available information, as well as the information relevant to the mental state examination (MSE) should be documented.

Appearance and behaviour The patient is dressed in a hospital gown; she is malodorous with unkempt hair. She avoids eye contact, and is suspicious and agitated.

Speech The patient gives inappropriate answers to your questions, with loosening of associations and sudden silences.

Mood She has an incongruous affect. It is not possible to establish whether there are any thoughts of harm to self or others.

Thoughts The patient appears to be thought disordered, with persecutory delusions and somatic hallucinations or passivity phenomena.

Perception She also appears to have auditory hallucinations.

Cognition At present it is not possible to assess her cognition because of the severity of her psychosis.

Insight The patient lacks insight. She is unable to provide informed consent for an admission and treatment.

Further history

Her brother, George, arrives at the hospital, allowing a collateral history to be obtained. He says that, looking back, she has not been 'quite right' for around a year, but has worsened considerably in the past two weeks, when she began to talk about hearing God and the Devil arguing about her.

A year ago she broke up with her fiancé. Soon after that she was made redundant from her role as a secretary. George comments that she did not put much effort into finding a new job, and has perhaps lost some of her normal sense of initiative. She has certainly lost interest in her personal appearance and housekeeping, and her neighbours have been complaining about her throwing flaming books from her window and playing 'hymns' at high volume day and night. She told a neighbour that the books were possessed by the Devil.

She has no previous psychiatric history, and, to the best of his knowledge, she has never taken illicit drugs. He is also unaware of any family history of mental illness.

Diagnostic approach

The patient has psychosis, with symptoms suggestive of schizophrenia: third person auditory hallucinations, passivity phenomena, thought disorder, a history of negative symptoms and a prodromal period. She requires further assessment and management in a psychiatric ward, which she is unable to provide informed consent for. As there is a considerable risk to her health and safety without a compulsory admission, a first medical recommendation admission under the relevant legislation (as she is in England, this is Section 2 of the Mental Health Act – see **Chapter 13**) is completed.

3.2 Schizophrenia

Schizophrenia is perhaps the archetypal psychiatric condition. It is a syndrome, encompassing a diverse range of often disabling symptoms, including hallucinations, delusions, disordered thinking and cognitive dysfunction. It is a major contributor to the global burden of disease owing to its early onset and often chronic course.

Despite the very real impact of its symptoms, the concept of schizophrenia is a controversial one. Schizophrenia is a circular

> Schizophrenia cannot be understood without understanding despair
>
> R. D. Laing

concept: it is defined by its constitutive symptoms; symptoms themselves defined according to the concept of schizophrenia.

There is no one pathognomonic feature, nor is there any specific investigation.

Some argue that the syndrome is unviable, as it does not coherently identify an underlying condition. These issues continue to be debated, as a continuation of the evolution of schizophrenia since it was first identified as a discrete syndrome in the nineteenth century.

Clinical insight

'Schizophrenia', from the ancient Greek for 'splitting of the mind'; not to be confused with the extremely rare and possibly non-existent multiple personality disorder.

Epidemiology

A person's lifetime risk of developing schizophrenia is thought to be around 1%. Estimates vary according to the diagnostic criteria used.

Men and women are generally affected in equal numbers, but men tend to have an earlier onset and more severe illness (possibly because of a lesser response to antipsychotics).

Schizophrenia most commonly presents in early adulthood:
- men: 15–25, with a mean of about 27 years
- women: 25–35, with a mean of about 32 years; women have a second, smaller, peak of onset around the time of menopause

Causes/pathogenesis

Schizophrenia is thought to be caused by a combination of genetic and environmental factors, specifically during brain development.

Genetics

Schizophrenia is strongly heritable. **Figure 3.1** shows the approximate risks associated with various family histories of schizophrenia. Adoption studies have shown that this increased risk is preserved in the children of parents with schizophrenia who are adopted by healthy parents.

At least 43 genes have been implicated in schizophrenia, including neuroregulin-1 and dysbindin. A number of genes contribute to an overall vulnerability to schizophrenia.

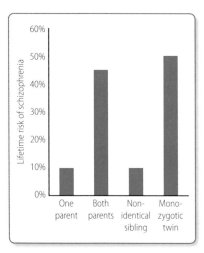

Figure 3.1 Lifetime risks of developing schizophrenia if there are affected relatives

Environmental

Perinatal and early childhood factors These include:
- maternal malnutrition/stress/infection
- obstetric complications
- having an older father
- being born in winter or spring – possibly a secondary effect of maternal infections
- delayed developmental milestones – particularly in the first year
- disturbed childhood behaviour
- early social services involvement

Immigration There is some indication that immigrants are over four times more likely to have schizophrenia than the native population. Afro-Caribbean immigrants to Europe, in particular, have

Clinical insight

People with schizophrenia have more significant life events in the weeks or months prior to admission than controls. Interpreting this correlation is difficult as the events could cause the onset/relapse of illness, or, inversely, the early prodromal/psychotic symptoms may lead to the events.

been the focus of much research, but the reason for this rise in rate remains unclear. Theories include:

- stressors associated with migration, such as the traumas being escaped
- bureaucratic problems
- difficulties integrating with the local population

Diagnostic bias by the local psychiatric services does not appear to be a significant factor.

Urabanicity/social factors Schizophrenia is twice as common in people living in an urban environment, with the highest admission rates in the most deprived areas. None of the possible explanations for this, such as the 'urban drift' of those with schizophrenia to cities, the 'social drift' of those with schizophrenia to lower socioeconomic classes, with pollution, overcrowding and infections, have been proven.

Clinical insight

In the 1950s it was noticed that the risk of a schizophrenia relapse was lower in people discharged to live alone than in those who returned to their partner or parents. Subsequent research has identified high amounts of a combination of overinvolvement, critical comments or hostility (referred to as high expressed emotion) from family members as a significant risk factor for relapse.

Cannabis use On average, marijuana users are 40% more likely to develop a psychotic illness, particularly if they start in adolescence. The risk increases with use.

Neurochemistry

Dopamine hypothesis This theory implicates excessive dopaminergic activity in the pathogenesis of schizophrenia:

- increased dopamine production or receptor sensitivity or number leads to symptoms
- positive symptoms (psychosis, excess or distorted normal functions) result from **raised** dopamine in the mesolimbic pathways (**Figure 3.2**)
- negative symptoms (loss or reduction of normal functions) are due to **lowered** dopamine in the mesocortical pathways

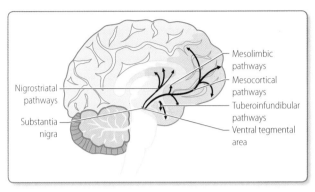

Figure 3.2 Dopaminergic pathways in the brain

Dopaminergic pathways include:
- **mesolimbic pathways**: ventral tegmental area (VTA) to the nucleus accumbens in the limbic system (positive symptoms)
- **mesocortical pathways**: VTA to the frontal cortex (negative symptoms)
- **nigrostriatal pathways**: substantia nigra to the striatum (extrapyramidal side-effects of antipsychotics)
- **tuberoinfundibular pathways**: hypothalamus to pituitary (antipsychotic-induced hyperprolactinaemia)

Evidence supporting the role of dopamine includes:
- all effective antipsychotic medications antagonise dopaminergic D_2 receptors
- amphetamines increase cerebral dopamine, and can cause psychosis

Glutamate hypothesis This hypothesis comes from the observation that phencyclidine (PCP) and ketamine block *N*-methyl-D-aspartate (NMDA)/glutamate receptors, and can cause psychosis.

Guiding principle

A **salience syndrome**: dopamine is involved in determining which stimuli we find important (salient). This may help to explain the basis of delusions and hallucinations. For instance, raised dopamine levels could lead a person to repeatedly find innocent objects such as passing police cars more personally significant than they really are.

NMDA/glutamate receptors seem to be involved in the regulation of dopamine release, suggesting that glutaminergic dysfunction underlies altered dopaminergic activity in schizophrenia.

Interestingly, in recent early clinical trials in patients with schizophrenia, a glutaminergic drug was found to perform as well as olanzapine.

Neuroanatomical changes

Specific abnormalities of cerebral structure have been associated with schizophrenia, including ventricular dilatation, and smaller prefrontal and temporal cortices, hippocampi and thalami. There also appear to be functional abnormalities of some of these areas.

Various histological abnormalities are also present, but no gliosis, which suggests that there is no neurodegenerative process.

> ## Clinical insight
>
> Remember the definition of a **delusion**: 'a fixed belief that is held in the face of evidence to the contrary, *not explained by culture or religion*'. Ideas thought to be delusional by some can be considered normal by others. For example, visions and voices may be a normal religious or spiritual experience in some cultures.

Clinical features

The key symptoms are separated into positive, negative and disorganised categories; cognitive and affective categories are also used (**Table 3.1**). Schizophrenia is largely diagnosed on the basis of particular psychotic symptoms, as reflected in the ICD-10 diagnostic criteria.

Schneider's first-rank symptoms

In 1959 Kurt Schneider proposed a set of 'first-rank' symptoms of schizophrenia to assist GPs with diagnosis. These classic symptoms are characterised by a transgression of the boundary between the person's internal world, and the external world. They are not diagnostic; around 20% of patients with schizophrenia have never had any first-rank symptoms, whereas 10% of non-schizophrenic patients have experienced at least one of them. Despite this, they still have influence on modern diagnostic criteria (and examination questions).

Symptoms	Clinical features
Positive (psychotic) symptoms Additional to normal experience, or exaggerated distortions of normal processes	Delusions
	Thought disorder
	Hallucinations
Negative symptoms Loss or reduction of normal functions	Anhedonia
	Flattened affect
	Apathy, avolition
	Social withdrawal
	Poverty of speech (alogia) and thought
	Poor self-care
Disorganised symptoms Noticeably chaotic or unpredictable behaviour that is not thought to be secondary to delusions	Poorly planned or purposeless actions
	Bizarre or silly behaviour
	Agitation
	Disinhibition
Cognitive symptoms Sometimes subtle abnormalities	Attention
	Learning
	Memory
	Executive function, e.g. planning and abstraction (overlap with disorganised symptoms)
Affective symptoms	Depression
	Anxiety
	Elation

Table 3.1 Clinical features of schizophrenia

Auditory hallucinations These include:
- **third person**: voices discuss the patient, e.g. 'he looks shifty'
- **running commentary**: voices comment on the patient's thoughts or actions
- **thought echo**: the patient's thoughts are heard spoken aloud. This is also known by the German *gedankenlautwerden*

('thoughts become loud'); can be thought of as a manifestation of the person's subjective loss of possession over their thoughts

Delusions of thought control (thought alienation) These include:
- **thought broadcast**: usually described as someone or something else having access to the patient's thoughts, often in the form of a secondary delusional elaboration (e.g. 'MI5 is reading my mind')
- **thought insertion**: usually described as someone or something else placing thoughts into the patient's mind; the insertion is thought to be a delusional explanation for the subjective experience of having thoughts over which the person has no control
- **thought withdrawal:** the opposite experience to thought insertion, this can be regarded as a delusional interpretation of **thought block** – when the mind is suddenly empty of thought (distinct from the sensation of being unable to think when anxious)

Passivity phenomena The person experiences a lack of control over aspects of their bodily functioning, again often producing a delusional explanation. These include:
- **somatic passivity:** the experience of someone or something else having control over the patient's bodily sensations
- **passivity of affect, volition, or impulse:** the experience of someone or something else having control over the patient's affect, volition or impulses

Delusional perception A normal percept is given a delusional significance.

Course of illness
The presentation, course and outcome of schizophrenia are different for every patient.

A **prodromal phase** often precedes the onset of schizophrenia. This includes subtle negative-type symptoms, strange thoughts and behaviours, anxiety, depression and preoccupations, which develop insidiously over a period of several years, and lead to deterioration in the patient's personal functioning

An **acute phase**, characterised by psychotic symptoms, typically brings the patient into contact with mental health services.

A **chronic** phase may follow the successful resolution of the acute phase, with negative and cognitive symptoms becoming prominent, and a risk of further relapses.

During the five years after a first episode:

- approximately 20% of patients recover and remain entirely well
- 35% have several further episodes with full recovery in between
- approximately 10% have several further episodes with stable impairment of baseline functioning in between
- approximately 35% have several further episodes with steadily increasing functional impairment

Approach to the patient

The patient with delusions

If the patient is profoundly psychotic with no insight, it may only be possible, because of thought disorder or hostility, to passively record their delusions. This information can be used later to assess improvements in insight. Asking about the origin of the beliefs may reveal important details such as contributory hallucinations, but, in some cases, this can be difficult.

If the patient is less unwell, then some careful challenges and exploratory questions may be appropriate. Asking for evidence in this way can provide a more subtle analysis of insight, as well

Clinical insight

Florid psychotic symptoms can be extremely distressing (e.g. the Devil taunting the patient or realistic somatic hallucinations of being raped) or pleasurable (e.g. hours in the company of singing angels).

Clinical insight

Acknowledge that the delusionary belief is important to the patient, without reinforcing it. Try to convey that you do not share the belief, but do not forcefully challenge it.

> ### Clinical insight
>
> Some patients spontaneously reveal their delusions, whereas others may be very guarded, speaking for a long time without evidence of illness.

as allowing a more intimate history and benefiting the therapeutic relationship.

Asking about delusions

It is sometimes useful to begin by stating that you need to ask some **routine** questions, which 'may seem a little odd':

• 'do you have any beliefs that other people find strange?'
• 'do you have any thoughts that other people don't share?'

Specific questions to identify delusions more common in schizophrenia are shown in **Table 3.2**.

Symptoms	Questions
Thought insertion or withdrawal, and thought broadcasting	'Are you able to think clearly?' 'Are your thoughts your own?' If no, ask how they know this, and determine where they feel that the thoughts come from 'Does it ever feel that someone or something is putting thoughts into/taking thoughts out of your head?' 'Can other people read your mind/access your thoughts?' 'Does it ever feel that your thoughts can be heard by others?'
Delusions of control, influence or passivity	'Is someone or something controlling you?' 'Is someone or something controlling your feelings/actions/sensations?' 'Has it ever felt that your movements/feelings/sensations are not yours?'
Delusions of reference	'Do people seem to be talking about you?' 'Do people seem to be signalling something to you?' 'Do people seem to be following you around?'
Delusions of persecution	'Do you feel safe?' 'Does it feel that someone is trying to harm you?'

Table 3.2 Example questions to identify delusions in schizophrenia

When delusions are cited in a referral, it may be better to explore delusional content through a general conversational history. For example, asking the patient what is troubling them may reveal fears about MI5 bugging their phone or their anxiety about aliens stealing their thoughts, which can then be explored further.

After eliciting some delusional content, ask the patient about other delusions common in schizophrenia. These questions can also be used as part of a complete mental state examination for other presenting complaints.

Asking about hallucinations

It may be helpful to start by saying: 'Stress can play tricks on people's imagination, such as causing them to hear voices when there is no one else there. Has this ever happened to you?'

Auditory or other hallucinations may be elicited indirectly in the history, such as the patient complaining about people in the street talking about them, or that they can feel a cat in their stomach.

Auditory hallucinations If voices are present, try to find out further details. For each voice, establish (qualities in the ICD-10 diagnostic criteria are shown in parentheses):

- where it comes from (coming from some part of the body)
- who it belongs to
- what it says
- its nature (a running commentary, discussion about the patient, thought echo)
- the patient's view on the voice; i.e. their insight into the hallucination
- the effect on the patient; is it distressing, can any commands be ignored?
- frequency
- duration

Other modalities Hallucinations in other modalities should be asked about:

- 'Have you ever seen anything unusual?'
- 'Have you ever had a vision?'
- 'Have you ever experienced a strange taste/smell without anything to cause it?'

- 'Have you ever had any strange sensations even though there seemed to be nothing to cause it?'

If present, determine their duration, and any accompanying delusions or overvalued thoughts.

Clinical insight

Remember that auditory hallucinations have a variety of possible causes, such as drugs, extreme stress, borderline personality disorder. They may also be hypnogogic/hypnopompic hallucinations (**Chapter 1**).

Hallucinations of the various senses, particularly those of smell and taste, can also be caused by temporal epilepsy.

Investigations

A first episode of psychosis necessitates a full physical (including neurological) examination. The following investigations should be carried out, both to help to rule out organic causes and to provide a baseline prior to potential antipsychotic treatment.

All patients should have the following assessments:
- full blood count (FBC)
- urea and electrolytes
- liver function tests
- thyroid function tests
- serum lipids
- fasting blood glucose
- weight and body mass index
- urine drug screen

Also, on a case-by-case basis:
- ECG, if there is a raised cardiovascular risk, or prior to the use of an antipsychotic with cardiovascular side-effects such as haloperidol
- cranial CT/MRI if, for example, a brain tumour is suspected
- urine dipstick test, to rule out a urinary tract infection
- pregnancy test, as this will affect management

Diagnostic criteria and differential diagnoses
ICD-10

At least one very clear symptom (or at least two if less clear-cut) from groups a–d below **or** symptoms from at least two of the groups e–h.

The symptoms must have been present for at least one month; if not, the diagnosis is **acute schizophrenia-like psychotic disorder**.

a. thought echo, insertion, withdrawal, or broadcast; delusions of control, influence or passivity; delusional perception
b. hallucinatory voices: running commentary on the patient's behaviour, discussing the patient among themselves, or coming from the body
c. persistent delusions of other kinds (completely impossible, e.g. being able to control the weather)
d. persistent hallucinations in any modality: accompanied by fleeting delusions without clear affective content, or by overvalued ideas, or occurring every day for weeks or months on end
e. breaks or interpolations in the train of thought
f. catatonic behaviour
g. 'negative' symptoms
h. a significant and consistent change in aspects of personal behaviour (loss of interest, aimlessness, idleness, a self-absorbed attitude and social withdrawal)

Subtypes

Various schizophrenia subtypes are recognised in the ICD-10 (see below). In practice, these are difficult to diagnose. The DSM-IV schizophrenia subtypes, which are very similar to those of the ICD-10, are proposed for deletion from the DSM-V.

Paranoid   This is the most common subtype. Delusions are the most prominent feature, often accompanied by hallucinations (usually auditory) and abnormal perceptions. Less common are disturbances of affect, volition and speech, or catatonic symptoms.

Hebephrenic   Alteration of affect is marked, with a shallow or inappropriate mood. There are often mannerisms. Behaviour is irresponsible and there is often social isolation. Thought is disordered, but delusions and hallucinations are less stable than in the paranoid type. Rapid development of negative symptoms leads to a poor prognosis.

Catatonic This subtype is now rare in developed countries, presumably secondary to antipsychotic use. It is characterised by psychomotor disturbances; from hyperkinesis and stupor to automatic obedience and negativism.

Undifferentiated Symptoms meet the schizophrenia diagnostic criteria, but do not clearly fit into any of the above subtypes.

Post-schizophrenic depression A depressive episode within a year of a schizophrenia relapse which confers an increased risk of suicide. Schizophrenic symptoms are confined to the background.

Residual Prominent negative symptoms mark a clear chronic phase of the illness. These symptoms are long term but not necessarily irreversible.

Simple A difficult and unreliable diagnosis, in which negative symptoms develop without prior overt psychosis.

Differential diagnosis

The differential diagnoses include organic psychosis, psychiatric conditions or other psychotic disorders.

Organic psychosis These include:

- drug-induced psychotic disorder, e.g. steroids, cannabis, cocaine, amphetamines, alcohol, L-dopa
- delirium
- dementia
- cerebral space-occupying lesion, infection or injury
- other neurological conditions, e.g. Wilson's or Huntington's disease
- Cushing's syndrome
- vitamin B_{12} deficiency
- tertiary syphilis
- systemic lupus erythematosus
- porphyria
- temporal lobe epilepsy

Psychiatric conditions These include:

- affective disorders: manic psychosis or psychotic depression
- puerperal psychosis
- personality disorders

Other psychotic disorders Those recognised by the ICD-10 are shown in **Table 3.3**.

Management

Pharmacological

Antipsychotic drugs (**Chapter 2**) effectively treat positive symptoms in around 80% of patients, although a short-term benzodiazepine or hypnotic may be required before they take full effect.

When choosing an antipsychotic, consider:

- current guidance does not recommend a first-line class or agent; consider the individual situation of the patient and carer(s)
- although clozapine is an effective second-generation antipsychotic, there is a 1% risk of potentially fatal agranulocytosis, which requires strict FBC monitoring. Thus it

Condition	Notes
Schizoaffective disorder	Affective and schizophrenic symptoms are both prominent in the same episode of illness and neither is particularly primary or predominant
Schizotypal disorder	There is unusual thinking, behaviour and affect, but the diagnostic criteria of schizophrenia are never met. It is classified as a personality disorder in DSM-IV
Persistent delusional disorder	This is characterised by a chronic delusion or set of related delusions, which may persist for life, and are not due to an organic, schizophrenic or affective condition
Acute and transient psychotic disorders	These are disorders characterised by non-organic acute psychosis and severely disturbed behaviour that may remit in days or within a few months at most, and include acute schizophrenia-like psychotic disorder

Table 3.3 Other psychotic conditions recognised by the ICD-10

is indicated only for **treatment-resistant schizophrenia** (the failed use of two antipsychotics, each trialled for six to eight weeks)
- **liquid** and orally dispersible antipsychotics may be useful in some cases, such as to prevent covert non-compliance (e.g. the patient spitting out tablets)
- **depot** or long-acting antipsychotics can be used to improve long-term adherence to medication. The most recent guidelines suggest offering these after the stabilisation of a first episode

Antipsychotics are usually be used for one to two years after a single episode.

Psychological

Current guidance recommends the following psychological therapies in schizophrenia, although unfortunately local resources vary considerably.
- **cognitive–behavioural therapy** in all patients. This has been shown to reduce the length of time spent in hospital, rehospitalisation rates, symptom severity and depression.
- **family intervention** to all families in close contact with the patient. This includes education about the condition and ways in which the family can support the patient. This has been reported to reduce relapse rate, hospital admissions and symptom severity.
- **arts therapy** to be considered in all patients. This has been found to be effective in reducing negative symptoms.

Social

The multidisciplinary team can provide assistance with issues such as employment, housing and benefits, as well as assessing the needs of any carers, children and vulnerable adults.

Clinical insight

Listening to music through headphones is a simple, cheap and empowering treatment for distressing auditory hallucinations

Complications/ prognosis

Although individual illness courses vary widely, and historical pessimism regarding the outcome has reduced, schizophrenia remains associated with significant morbidity and economic cost.

Key factors affecting prognosis are shown in **Table 3.4**.

Morbidity and mortality

High rates of smoking, poor diet, lack of exercise and antipsychotic use make people with schizophrenia at increased risk of chronic health problems such as cardiovascular disease and type 2 diabetes; physical health should be monitored yearly. Tests should include fasting blood glucose, weight/body mass index and blood pressure, as well as assessment of smoking, alcohol and drug use. Monitoring should also consider side-effects of antipsychotic use.

Life expectancy is reduced in schizophrenia, for example by ten years in the UK. Most deaths result from chronic medical conditions, such as cardiovascular disease.

The suicide rate for people with schizophrenia is around 7%, and accounts for half of all deaths by age 39. The risk of suicide is highest in the first year, and is increased by:

- social isolation
- depression
- unemployment

There are also significant social problems associated with schizophrenia, including:

- unemployment
- homelessness

Worse prognosis	Better prognosis
Male gender	Good premorbid adjustment
Longer duration of untreated illness	Acute onset
Early or insidious onset	Older age at onset
Substance misuse	Prominent positive symptoms
Negative symptoms	Prominent affective symptoms
Family history of schizophrenia	Being married
Social isolation	Having good social/family support
Lower social class	Good response to medication
Extensive psychiatric history	Compliance with medication
High expressed emotion	

Table 3.4 Factors affecting schizophrenia prognosis

- involvement in the criminal justice system
- substance misuse

Stigma

The stigma of schizophrenia can be more distressing than the symptoms themselves. It can also precipitate or exacerbate social isolation, substance misuse, unemployment, institution-alisation and homelessness.

Attitudes can be changed. For example, in 2002 the Japanese term for schizophrenia, *seishin-bunretsu-byo* (mind-split disease), was changed to *togo-shitcho-sho* (integration disorder). There is evidence of a subsequent reduction in both stigma-tisation and the general public's association of schizophrenia with violence.

Affective (mood) disorders

chapter

4

4.1 Clinical scenario

A decline in mood following a manic episode

Presentation

Caitlin is a 47 year old lady who was discharged to the home treatment service from a psychiatric ward two months ago, following treatment for a first manic episode. She had been admitted following her arrest for attempting to adopt the children of strangers. The plan was for her to be discharged this week to the community mental health team, but concerns have been raised about her declining mood.

Previous psychiatric history

At her initial admission, she had been extravagantly dressed, and carried a list of 'her' children's names. Restless, and occasionally flirtatious, she had communicated with loud, pressured and circumstantial speech. She was clearly elated, sometimes irritable, with mood-congruent delusions of grandeur. Her thoughts had sometimes been difficult to follow because of her flight of ideas, but they revolved around her being 'blessed by God with 100 children', the names of whom had been communicated directly to her by the Angel Gabriel. She had been stopped in the process of collecting the children in order to take them 'to live at Stonehenge', where she would 'rule as Queen'.

She presented a risk to others and lacked insight into her illness, and was admitted under Section 2 of the Mental Health Act (England and Wales) for further assessment.

Diagnostic approach

Due to a lack of known contacts, no collateral history was available. As this appeared to be her first presentation, she was fully investigated for organic causes, none of which were found. She had recovered well with antipsychotic medication.

Today, Caitlin's mental state needs to be reviewed, and her need for continued home treatment team (HTT) input should be assessed. Are there any risks to others, such as children? If she is depressed, what is the severity, and are there any thoughts of self-harm?

Initial history

She opens the door after a prolonged wait, and appears unkempt. The flat is untidy, although not dirty. Her movements are not slow, but she does not maintain eye contact and her facial expressions are limited.

She reports that she has not been well over the past week, lacking in energy and spending most of the time in bed. She used to enjoy visiting the market, but this no longer interests her. She also complains of a headache and joint pains.

She states that she is unsure why she has gone downhill, but later mentions feeling isolated and lonely. Becoming slightly tearful, she describes feeling that she has failed in life, as she has not married and raised a family, like 'normal people do'.

Diagnostic approach

Caitlin appears depressed, so other common symptoms of depression should be inquired about.

Further history

Caitlin is sleeping poorly, tending to wake in the early hours, and her appetite is reduced, although she manages to eat sufficiently. Her motivation is reduced, and she finds it difficult to concentrate on long TV programmes.

She feels pessimistic about the future, and views herself as a failure. She admits to vague thoughts 'in the back of my mind' of 'not wanting to wake up', but denies any plans to self-harm, as this would be against her Christian beliefs. She has no thoughts of harming others, or regarding 'adopting' children.

No evidence of hypomania/mania, anxiety or psychosis is found. She also denies the use of alcohol or drugs.

Further investigation into her physical symptoms indicates that there are no underlying medical conditions. She agrees with the suggestion that these symptoms are related to her low mood.

Diagnostic approach

A full history and mental state examination need to be completed. The impression at this point is that Caitlin has bipolar affective disorder, and is currently presenting with symptoms of a moderate depressive episode. There is a low risk of harm to herself and others at present.

Following discussion within the HTT, it is decided that she needs continued support from the team for further treatment and monitoring. Her medication will be reviewed, with consideration given to antidepressants (with caution so as to avoid the precipitation of hypomania/mania) and mood stabilisers. In addition, the team occupational therapist will look into organising some social activities.

> ## Guiding principle
>
> In affective disorders there are changes of mood in excess to those experienced in normal life. These changes may be:
>
> - **unipolar:** an abnormally depressed mood only
> - **bipolar:** both depression and an abnormally elevated mood

4.2 Depression

The features of normal sadness, known to everybody, are magnified and transformed in depression. The low mood is stubbornly persistent; normal interests and reactivity of mood fade away; and negative thoughts of hopelessness and guilt are painful preoccupations. Debilitating physical symptoms, such as insomnia, anorexia and loss of libido, may be predominant.

> I am in that temper that if I were under water I would scarcely kick to come to the top.
>
> John Keats

According to the World Health Organization, depression was the fourth leading contributor to the worldwide burden of disease in 2000. By 2020, it is projected to rise to second place worldwide, and to become the most significant cause of disability in the developed world.

Epidemiology

Depression is the most common psychiatric disorder in the UK, with a lifetime risk in the general population of approximately 15%.

Women are almost twice as commonly affected as men. The reasons for this may include:

- genetic and hormonal differences
- pregnancy and childbirth
- sociocultural roles with an increased risk of adverse circumstances
- higher reporting rates and diagnostic bias by doctors

Depression can affect people of any age, although peak onsets are old age in men and middle age in women.

Guiding principle

There are variations in the prevalence of depression around the world. This is probably related, at least partly, to the sometimes dramatic differences in the presentation of depression between cultures.

For example, African and Asian people commonly present with **somatic symptoms**, e.g. aches and pains. This may be due to the influence of cultural backgrounds with little recognition of depression; and a conscious, or unconscious, fear of the stigma of mental illness. Patients may anticipate a more comfortable consultation with conventional symptoms, or perhaps presume that a doctor will be more interested in, and tolerant of, a physical complaint.

Causes/pathogenesis

Historically there has been much debate surrounding a supposed difference between a biological or **endogenous** depression, which:

- had a genetic basis
- produced somatic symptoms
- was independent of life events

and a neurotic or **reactive** depression, which:

- was affected by environmental factors
- presented in a number of forms
- ran a variable course

Nowadays, depression is considered to result from complex interactions of biological, psychological and social factors.

Genetics

There is a genetic component to depression:

- first-degree relatives of a person with depression are at increased risk
- concordance rates in monozygotic twins are 46% compared with 20% in dizygotic twins
- adoption studies have shown that children of parents with depression retain their increased risk when living in unaffected families
- the inheritance is likely to be polygenic, along with complex environmental interactions

Environmental

Life events   There may be an excess of life events in the two to three months prior to an episode of depression. Loss is a key theme of such life events:

- the most significant event is the death of a spouse
- divorce or separation
- imprisonment
- death of a close relative
- unemployment
- home relocation

Childhood   Factors that increase the risk of depression include:

- the loss of a parent without an adequate replacement
- childhood sexual abuse
- poor parental care, such as excess criticism and a lack of affection

Social   Factors associated with depression include:

- lower socioeconomic status
- social isolation
- not being married
- unemployment

Clinical insight

Interestingly, there are gender differences with some social factors. In women, the lack of a confiding relationship is a particularly important risk factor; and in men, separation or divorce. Also, men gain more of a protective benefit from marriage than do women.

Psychological

Cognitive theories These emphasise the contribution of an individual's interpretation of stressful events. Some researchers point to how maladaptive cognitive patterns, which lead to excessively negative interpretations, originate from negative experiences in the past.

A key cognitive theory involves **Beck's triad**, which describes three types of negative thoughts held by a depressed person:

- the self (e.g. 'I'm useless')
- the present (e.g. 'I hate my job')
- the future (e.g. 'I feel hopeless')

Personality traits Neuroticism, anxiety, impulsivity and obsessional traits may predispose to depression, whereas a relaxed temperament offers some protection.

Organic

Chronic, severe and painful physical illnesses are particularly likely to lead to depression.

Medical causes of depression include:

- cancer
- cardiovascular disease
- neurological disease (e.g. multiple sclerosis, Parkinson's disease, stroke, epilepsy)
- endocrine disease (e.g. diabetes, Cushing's syndrome, hypothyroidism, hyperparathyroidism, hypercalcaemia)
- infective disease (e.g. human immunodeficiency virus (HIV)/ acquired immunodeficiency syndrome, infectious mononucleosis, hepatitis)
- metabolic disease (e.g. vitamin B_{12}/folate deficiency, iron deficiency)
- drugs: substance abuse (e.g. alcohol, steroids, cannabis, cocaine)

- medication (e.g. steroids, beta blockers, calcium channel blockers, digoxin, opioids, methyldopa)

Neurochemical

Monoamine hypothesis This theory suggests that depression results from a reduction in the activity of monoamine neurotransmitters, such as serotonin (5-hydroxytryptamine; 5HT), dopamine, noradrenaline and adrenaline. There may be an absolute reduction in the amount of monoamines, or a relative reduction from lowered receptor activity. Evidence supporting this hypothesis is given in **Table 4.1**.

The monoamine theory is now felt to be oversimplistic, not least from research showing that other neurotransmitter systems (e.g. γ-aminobutyric acid (GABA) and acetylcholine) can be altered in depression. A contemporary theory suggests there is a reduction in **neurotrophic factors** in depression, leading to abnormal functioning and death of neurones, particularly in the hippocampus.

Endocrine

Neuroendocrine dysfunction causing stress or endocrine disease is associated with depression and bipolar disorder.

Stress This has various important effects on the body (see **Chapter 7**), including alterations in brain function. Such effects are predominantly mediated through cortisol-releasing hormone (CRH) and the hypothalamic–pituitary–adrenal (HPA) axis.

Drug	Effect
Reserpine	Decreases monoamine activity and can lead to depression
Amphetamines and cocaine	Increase monoamines and can elevate the mood
Antidepressants	Increase monoamine levels

Table 4.1 Evidence for the monoamine hypothesis.

Endocrine diseases Cushing's syndrome, Addison's disease and thyroid problems can all feature depression.

Evidence There is some evidence for **endocrinological dysfunction** in depression. For example, there is increased activity of the hypothalamic–pituitary–adrenal axis in depressed patients, as determined by:
- higher concentrations of cortisol-releasing hormone in the cerebrospinal fluid (CSF)
- non-suppression of cortisol by dexamethasone

The hypothalamic–pituitary–thyroid axis changes in depressed patients, as determined by:
- raised thyroid-releasing factor (TRF) in the CSF
- attenuated thyroid-stimulating hormone response to TRF challenge

Neuroanatomical

Inconsistent findings of enlarged lateral ventricles and a reduction in the volumes of the frontal and temporal lobes, hippocampus and basal ganglia have been reported in depression.

Immunological

The reported changes in depression include increased proinflammatory cytokines and acute-phase proteins, and reduced T-cell replication and natural killer cell activity.

Clinical features

The symptoms of depression are shown in **Table 4.2**.
Depression can present with atypical features, such as:
- mood reactivity
- increased appetite (hyperphagia)
- increased sleep (hypersomnia)
- personality issues, with resultant history of rejection by others
- increased anxiety in some patients

Course of illness

Depressive episodes usually last for 3–8 months. The majority are mild, with many spontaneously resolving before

Type	Symptoms
Core symptoms	**Depressed mood:** there may be diurnal variation (usually worse in the mornings)
	Anhedonia: inability to enjoy previously pleasurable experiences, with a loss of interest in work or pastimes
	Anergia: reduced energy and easy fatigability. The patient may be 'tired all the time'
Psychological symptoms	**Poor concentration and attention**
	Pessimism
	Low self-esteem
	Feelings of guilt
	Thoughts of self-harm and suicide
	Anxiety
	Poor memory
	Poor motivation
Somatic/biological symptoms	**Disturbed sleep:** early morning waking (2 or more hours early)/initial insomnia (difficulty getting to sleep)
	Decreased appetite: and possible weight loss
	Reduced libido
	Constipation
	Aches and pains
	Psychomotor disturbance: agitation or retardation (usually in more severe depression)
Bold text denotes use in ICD-10 diagnostic criteria.	

Table 4.2 Symptoms of depression

being detected. The remainder of patients (around one-third) experience moderate or severe symptoms.

The likelihood of recurrence after a severe first depressive episode is 80%; if less severe, it is around 50%. The risk of recurrence subsequently increases with each relapse. Most people recover well in between episodes, but about 20% develop chronic depression, especially those in later life.

Approach to the patient

People with depression should be approached sensitively:

- try to ask open questions and be patient
- allow the person time to express what may be difficult feelings to articulate
- listen carefully, making it clear that you are doing so with simple verbal acknowledgements, or physical cues such as nodding your head
- do not be judgemental, make easy assumptions or offer facile suggestions

The way patients recount their story may offer some insight into the causes of their problems; for example, from the way they talk about relationships, the emphasis they place on certain factors, and their cognitions and feelings in reaction to particular situations.

Clinical insight

Body language: mirroring the depressed patient is a powerful way of putting them at ease and establishing rapport. Adopt, for example, their soft, slow speech, and, if they appear withdrawn in their questions and body language, avoid being intrusive or hectoring.

Transference

Patients may elicit in you a variety of feelings during interviews. This **transference** may not be positive but can often be useful in gaining insight into patients. For example, it can help you better understand their difficulties with interpersonal relationships, or the negative reaction of their family to the illness, as well as teaching you something about yourself.

Questioning

Initial questioning Simple enquiries about a low mood include:

- 'How has your mood been recently?'
- 'Are there times when you feel low or tearful?'
- 'Have you been feeling reasonably cheerful recently?'

Further questioning If there seems to be a problem with a low mood, ask about other core, and common, symptoms from the clinical features section; for example,

- 'How have you been spending your days recently?'
- 'Do you still enjoy doing things as you used to?'
- 'How are your energy levels/do you sometimes struggle to find the energy or motivation to do things?'
- 'Has your concentration been affected … perhaps when reading the newspaper or watching TV etc.?'
- 'How has your sleep/appetite/sex drive been recently?'
- 'Do you have difficulty falling asleep/do you find yourself waking up in the early hours?'
- 'Have you lost weight recently … perhaps you've noticed your clothes are looser than usual?'
- 'What do you feel that the future holds?'
- 'Do you feel that life is worth living?'

For suicide risk assessment, see **Chapter 5**.

Psychosis

Is there any evidence of psychosis? Possible questions to use when enquiring about delusions include the following.

Delusions of guilt Ask patients:
- 'Do you feel you as though you have committed a crime/sinned/deserve to be punished?'
- 'Do you have any regrets?'

Nihilistic delusions Ask patients:
- 'Do you feel that something terrible has happened or is going to happen?'
- 'Do you feel as though you have died?'
- 'Do you feel that a part of your body has stopped working/is no longer there?'

Investigations

There are no specific investigations for depression. Tests may be required to rule out organic causes or as a baseline prior to pharmacological treatment, on a case-by-case basis. These may include full blood count, urea and electrolytes, liver function tests, thyroid-stimulating hormone, calcium, vitamin B_{12} and folate, erythrocyte sedimentation rate, HIV screening, and brain imaging.

Diagnostic criteria and differential diagnoses
ICD-10 criteria

The ICD-10 requires the presence of symptoms for at least two weeks, unless they are very severe.

Episodes of depression are classified in severity according to the number of other common symptoms (indicated by bold in **Table 4.2**) accompanying the core symptoms.

The first episode would be recorded as a mild, moderate or severe depressive episode, whereas any further episodes would be termed **recurrent depressive disorder**; current episode mild, moderate or severe.

Mild depression This is the commonest form and is often seen by GPs, although many patients may not present to a doctor at all. Coexistent anxiety is common.

> ### Guiding principle
>
> Many people with depression present with symptoms other than a low mood, such as feeling tired all the time, poor sleep or a low libido. They may be irritable rather than tearful. Neither ICD-10 nor DSM-IV requires low mood in order for a diagnosis of depression to be made.

ICD-10 criteria include:
- at least two core symptoms, plus at least two other symptoms
- none of the symptoms present to an intense degree

Moderate depression This is 'text book depression'; it is often treated in primary care, but may necessitate psychiatric input.

ICD-10 criteria include:
- at least two core symptoms, plus at least three other symptoms
- usually significant difficulties with social, work and domestic functioning

Severe depression Intense symptoms lead to a significant risk of self-neglect and suicide. Psychomotor retardation may progress to stupor and subsequent dehydration, malnutrition and bedsores. Electroconvulsive therapy (ECT) may be the only life-saving option.

The **ICD-10** separates severe depression into those with (10–25%) and those without psychotic symptoms.

DSM-IV criteria

The DSM-IV uses the term '**major depressive disorder**' for clinically significant depression. This can be classified as a single episode or recurrent, and all episodes require a minimum of five core symptoms from a list similar to that of the ICD-10. At least one symptom must be depressed mood or a loss of interest or pleasure.

Severity, as in ICD-10, is graded as mild, moderate or severe; however, in DSM-IV, this is based on the degree of social/occupational impairment.

Differential diagnoses

The differential diagnoses include:

- normal sadness
- seasonal affective disorder (see below)
- adjustment disorder, grief reaction (see below)
- anxiety disorder
- emotionally unstable personality disorder
- bipolar affective disorder
- negative symptoms of schizophrenia
- schizoaffective disorder
- extrapyramidal side-effects of antipsychotics
- dysthymia (see below)
- eating disorder
- organic disease (see causes)

Seasonal affective disorder In SAD episodes of depression recur at similar times each year (usually from winter to spring), and are marked by

> ## Clinical insight
>
> Psychotic symptoms in depression:
>
> - are classically **mood congruent**, revolving around themes, e.g. death, sin, guilt, poverty and catastrophe
> - may manifest in persecutory or nihilistic delusions, auditory hallucinations of derogatory voices or olfactory hallucinations of rotting flesh
>   - auditory hallucinations are usually brief and in the second person, distinguishing them from those of classic schizophrenia
>   - visual hallucinations are more rare, and should lead to consideration of an organic causation
>
> **Cotard's syndrome** is a rare presentation of psychotic depression; the person has nihilistic/somatic delusions, leading them to believe they are dead, non-existent, decaying or lacking their organs or blood.

atypical symptoms such as weight gain. A minority of people may experience hypomanic symptoms in spring/summer.

Dysthymia Also referred to as 'persistent subthreshold depressive symptoms', this consists of at least two years of subthreshold depressive symptoms. It is a common affliction, with an estimated lifetime prevalence of 2.5–5%. The majority of patients eventually meet the diagnostic criteria for depression.

Bereavement and grief Grief reaction is included in adjustment disorders in the ICD-10 (see **Chapter 7**). It is a normal reaction to loss, and should not be treated as a medical condition unless the symptoms are:

- delayed
- particularly severe
- persist for over 6 months

In contrast to depression, the distress tends to fluctuate and be concentrated on the loss, without pervading other aspects of life. Somatic symptoms such as poor sleep and appetite may occur, but anhedonia and cognitions of hopelessness, guilt and worthlessness point to depression.

Management
Antidepressant medication

Antidepressants are no better than placebo for mild depression. They are more effective in treating moderate to severe for which short-term trials (4–12 weeks) show a 50–60% response rate compared with a 30% response rate to placebo.

Choice of antidepressant Selective serotonin reuptake inhibitors (SSRIs) are usually used initially, but the particular choice of antidepressant should be made in conjunction with the patient, and take into account the following factors:

- previous effective use (take into account the patient's **perception** of this)
- potential side-effects and discontinuation syndromes
- potential interactions with current medication (citalopram has fewer interactions; fluoxetine more)

- suicidality (tricyclic antidepressants are most toxic in overdose)
- pregnancy and breast-feeding (see **Chapter 2**)

Prescribing antidepressants

Regularly monitor the patient. If there is no response after three to four weeks, and the patient is taking the medication as prescribed, the dose may be increased, or an alternative antidepressant used.

Initially, another SSRI or a newer generation antidepressant can be tried; subsequently, a less well-tolerated class may be considered.

In some cases, antidepressants may be augmented with other agents, such as lithium, an antipsychotic or another antidepressant such as mirtazapine.

- An effective antidepressant should be continued for at least 6 months after remission to reduce the risk of relapse
- If there remains a high risk of relapse after this, e.g. because of continued psychosocial stressors or a long history of recurrences, it should be continued for a further two years

> **Clinical insight**
>
> Treatment concordance with antidepressants can be poor. A strong patient–doctor relationship and psychoeducation can help to improve this.

> **Clinical insight**
>
> Antidepressants are not addictive, but patients should be warned about the so-called 'withdrawal' effects that constitute **antidepressant discontinuation syndrome**:
>
> - restlessness
> - sweating
> - unusual symptoms, e.g. paraesthesia
> - insomnia
> - unsteadiness
> - abdominal discomfort
> - mood changes
>
> Symptoms are usually mild and self-limiting, lasting around a week, but can be severe. Paroxetine causes most symptoms, owing to its short half-life; the converse is true of fluoxetine.
>
> A slow down-titration of the dose can help; however, this can prolong symptoms, so some clinicians recommend more abrupt cessation.
>
> It is important to distinguish between discontinuation syndrome and relapse of depression.

Psychological interventions

Psychological therapies for depressive symptoms include the following.

For **mild depression and dysthymia**:

- guided self-help
- computerised cognitive–behavioural therapy (CBT)
- peer support groups
- structured physical activity groups

For **moderate to severe depression**:

- individual or group CBT
- interpersonal psycho-therapy
- couples therapy

For **relapse prevention**:

- individual CBT
- mindfulness-based cognitive therapy; involving:
  - improving the understanding of depression
  - identifying personal vulnerability factors, including excessive self-imposed pressure to meet the perceived standards of society
  - subsequent blinding to what makes life worthwhile

In addition, befriending programmes and social rehabilitation may be useful for some people.

Clinical insight

Some believe that both doctors and patients rely too heavily on antidepressants. Patients with depression are likely to have complex psychosocial problems, extending beyond abnormal monoamine function. An effective management strategy may include antidepressants, but their efficacy is not beyond question.

Meta-analyses and study of data unpublished by drug companies reveal that many benefits are also provided by placebos. Such publishing bias can also obscure potential harm. Eyding et al. (2010) found that published data on reboxetine, a selective noradrenaline reuptake inhibitor, overestimated its benefit versus placebo and selective serotonin reuptake inhibitors by up to 115% and 23%, respectively, while also underestimating harm.

Complications/prognosis

The risk factors for a worse prognosis include:

- a more severe initial episode
- earlier onset
- a higher amount of required treatment
- psychiatric or physical comorbidities

Depression has important personal, social and economic ramifications; namely, it:

- contributes to a significant loss in quality of life, affecting relationships, family and employment

- increases the morbidity and mortality of physical disorders, such as cardio-vascular disease
- is associated with substance misuse
- increases the risk of suicide to four times that of the general population; those with more severe illness are at greater risk

> **Clinical insight**
>
> The risk that someone with recurrent depression will develop mania or hypomania never disappears.

4.3 Bipolar disorder

The occurrence of manic (or milder hypomanic) episodes distinguishes bipolar disorder from depression. Significant mood disturbances are interspersed with periods of improvement, the pattern noted by Kraepelin when he separated 'manic–depressive psychosis' from schizophrenia.

> I am excessively slothful, and wonderfully industrious – by fits. There are epochs when any kind of mental exercise is torture … I have thus rambled and dreamed away whole months, and awake, at last, to a sort of mania for composition. Then I scribble all day, and read all night, so long as the disease endures.
>
> Edgar Allen Poe

The DSM-IV divides bipolar disorder into types I and II, cyclothymia and rapid cycling (**Table 4.3**).

Epidemiology
The lifetime prevalence of bipolar disorder is approximately 1%.

Bipolar disorder usually begins between early adolescence and the early twenties.

Men and women are generally equally affected, although type II may be more common in women.

Causes/pathogenesis
Genetics
Genetics play a significant role in bipolar disorder. The risk of first-degree relatives of an

> **Clinical insight**
>
> Up to one-fifth of patients (many with a history of depression) are only diagnosed with bipolar disorder after the age of 50. There is some suggestion that this subgroup is genetically distinct from those with an earlier onset.

Classification	Description
Bipolar I	Marked by intense manic, or mixed manic and depressive, episodes. The depressive episodes between manic episodes are usually also severe
Bipolar II	Marked by hypomanic episodes, in which the symptoms are insufficiently severe to meet the criteria for mania
Rapid cycling	Used to describe the 10% of bipolar disorder type I or II in which there are more than four mood swings within a year
Cyclothymia	Consists of fluctuations in mood below the threshold of bipolar disorder. People with cyclothymia may go on to develop bipolar disorder

Table 4.3 Bipolar disorder classification in DSM-IV

Clinical insight

There appears to be an overlap in the genetics of unipolar depression and bipolar disorder, as the risk of major depression is doubled in first-degree relatives of people with bipolar disorder.

affected individual developing bipolar disorder is increased to 5–10%, and the concordance in monozygotic twins is around 60%. The inheritance is likely to be multigenic.

Psychosocial influences

The following psychological and social factors are associated with bipolar disorder:
- childhood maltreatment may increase the risk, perhaps by affecting the HPA axis and thus response to stress
- adverse life situations can act as triggers for episodes; such stressors may relate to social class, level of social support and self-esteem, and might partially explain the high levels of bipolar disorder in ethnic minority groups
- high expressed emotion (see **Chapter 3**) increases the risk of depressive episodes

Organic

Organic factors associated with bipolar disorder include:
- sleep deprivation

- childbirth
- endocrine: thyroid disorders, Cushing's syndrome
- neurological: cerebrovascular disease, cerebral space-occupying lesions, multiple sclerosis, epilepsy, head injuries
- drugs: antidepressants, corticosteroids, thyroid hormones, L-dopa, alcohol, stimulants

Neuroendocrinological

As with depression and anxiety disorders, neuroendocrine abnormalities appear to play a key role. The hypothalamic–pituitary–thyroid axis may be particularly important in bipolar disorder, especially in rapid cycling disorder.

> ### Clinical insight
>
> The idea of **manic defence** is that features of mania, such as grandiosity, are an overcompensating avoidance of negative cognitions, such as low self-worth, which are damaging to the ego.

Structural brain differences

Frontal and temporal lobe abnormalities in people with bipolar disorder have been suggested.

Clinical features

Depressive symptoms

The depressive symptoms are identical to those in unipolar depression.

Manic symptoms

From DSM-IV, these are:

- elevated/expansive/irritable mood
- inflated self-esteem/grandiosity
- distractibility
- increase in goal-directed activity/psychomotor agitation
- excessive participation in gratifying activities without consideration of the consequences, such as shopping sprees, sexual indiscretions or business investments
- flight of ideas
- more talkative than usual
- decreased need for sleep

A lack of insight is also characteristic of manic episodes.

Clinical insight

Psychotic symptoms in mania are usually mood congruent, such as delusions of grandeur or religious delusions. For example, the patient may believe that he is the Second Coming of Jesus, perhaps also hearing the voices of angels back in Heaven. Persecutory delusions also occur in mania.

Mixed episode

It is fairly common for patients to present with symptoms of both depression and mania. Depression is usually predominant, and suicide risk is increased.

Hypomanic episode

This is a milder presentation of a manic episode, in which the mood disturbance does not lead to marked impairment and there are no psychotic symptoms.

Course of illness

Manic episodes usually have an acute onset and, if untreated, tend to last three to six months. Depressive episodes persist longer, for around six months to a year if untreated.

The frequency of relapses increases with age.

Many people have subthreshold depression between manic or depressive episodes, rather than having periods of full remission.

Approach to the patient

People in a manic state can be challenging to interview, as they may be:

- preoccupied with recounting their achievements in great detail
- uninterested in your insignificant questions
- flirtatious, even tactile
- suspicious and scared

Patients' thoughts may race from topic to topic, making it difficult to understand and to interrupt; attempts to break the flow of their speech, which is probably rapid and loud, may trigger anger and aggression. Their simmering irritability may accompany drops into despair and leaps into elation, and their exasperation at your apparent shortcomings may be unashamedly displayed. On the other hand, the transfer to you of a patient's enthusiasm and elation can be enjoyable.

Safety and boundaries

Personal safety is the most important factor, so keep in mind the points mentioned in **Chapter 1**.

Manic patients can be unpredictable, with a fluctuating mood that may swing unexpectedly to anger, aggression and even violence. Disinhibition may lead to inappropriate verbal and physical behaviour.

Establishing boundaries is crucial. A delicate balance needs to be achieved between gathering the history and allowing patients to express themselves. Keeping a patient with tangential, pressured speech focused may require confident, forceful interruptions, but take care not to inflame tensions by being excessively restrictive.

Questioning

Initial questioning Good initial questions to use when enquiring about an elevated/expansive mood include:
- 'Have you sometimes felt particularly cheerful?'
- 'Have you been feeling on top of the world?'

Further questioning If there seems to be an elevated mood, ask about other key symptoms:
- 'Have you felt full of energy recently?'
- 'Do you feel that your mind is racing or that you have had lots of thoughts or ideas lately?'
- 'Do you need less sleep than usual?'
- 'Have you been spending more money than usual/have you bought anything interesting recently?'

Delusions of grandeur Enquire about delusions of grandeur:
- 'Do you have any exciting plans at the moment?'
- 'How would you compare yourself to other people?'
- 'Do you feel that you have any special abilities/powers/talents?'
- 'Do you feel you have a special mission?'
- 'Do you know anybody famous/any royalty?'
- 'Are you famous/prestigious/royalty?'
- 'Are you particularly close to God?'

Investigations

When carrying out investigations:

- precipitating physical conditions should be sought with a physical examination; urine dipstick and drug screen; and routine blood tests, including a full blood count and thyroid function tests

> ## Clinical insight
>
> An outlandish statement may not represent a delusion. A person with strong religious beliefs, for example, may talk of receiving God's Word, or of being possessed by a demon. These beliefs may be metaphorical statements rather than indications of psychopathology.

- baseline results of basic blood tests are also useful if medication is to be used
- brain imaging and other investigations may be indicated on a case-by-case basis

Diagnostic criteria and differential diagnoses
ICD-10

A diagnosis of bipolar disorder requires at least two episodes of significant mood disturbance, one of which must be mania or hypomania.

Episodes can be specified as:
- hypomanic
- manic without psychotic symptoms
- manic with psychotic symptoms
- mild or moderate depression
- severe depression without psychotic symptoms
- severe depression with psychotic symptoms
- mixed
- in remission

ICD-10 does not separate bipolar into types I and II.

DSM-IV

Manic episode This is a well-defined period of persistently and abnormally elevated, expansive or irritable mood, accompanied by at least three of the symptoms listed in the clinical features (four if the mood is only irritable).

The symptoms should have been present for at least one week (less if admission to hospital is required) and sufficiently severe to cause marked impairment in functioning/require admission to hospital/consist of psychosis.

Bipolar I This is defined as at least one manic or mixed episode.

Bipolar II This consists of at least one major depressive episode and at least one hypomanic episode. A manic or mixed episode changes the diagnosis to bipolar I.

Cyclothymia This is defined as at least two years of mood fluctuations that cause significant functional impairment; these may be sub- or full-threshold hypomanic episodes, and subthreshold depressive periods.

Differential diagnosis
The differential diagnoses include:
- organic conditions (see Causes)
- other psychiatric conditions, such as schizoaffective disorder; schizophrenia; and psychotic depression

Recent UK research in primary care (Smith et al., 2011) has shown that up to one-fifth of patients with depression may have unrecognised bipolar disorder. There is no reliable way to predict whether depression will develop into bipolar disorder, but the following are pointers:
- family history of bipolar disorder, especially a first-degree relative
- younger onset
- severe anhedonia
- feelings of worthlessness
- atypical depression
- psychomotor retardation
- psychotic features
- poor response to antidepressants

Management
People with mania rarely have insight into their condition. It is perhaps not surprising that a person who believes themselves

to be the Saviour of the World does not believe that they are unwell.

The behaviour of people with mania may put themselves or others at risk, and compulsory admission and treatment can sometimes be the only option. Hypomanic symptoms may be more easily managed in a community setting.

A short-term benzodiazepine use is useful for agitation and behavioural disturbance.

ECT is used in rare cases to treat severe symptoms that do not respond to other treatments.

Pharmacological

Acute episodes For further details of the pharmacological treatment of acute episodes, see **Table 4.4**.

Long-term prophylactic treatment The indications for long-term prophylactic treatment are:
- one significant manic episode
- two or more manic episodes
- frequent episodes in bipolar disorder type II
- a high risk of suicide
- significant functional impairment

The recommended medications are lithium, olanzapine and valproate, in combination if needed. Lamotrigine or carbamazepine may also be added later.

Prophylactic treatment should continue for at least two years after an episode, or for up to five years if risk factors for relapse are present (see Prognosis).

People who have chronic or recurrent depressive episodes, without a recent manic episode, and who are not prescribed prophylaxis may be given long-term selective serotonin reuptake inhibitors, quetiapine or lamotrigine (especially if bipolar disorder type II).

Psychological

Psychoeducation, especially about relapse indicators, is a crucial intervention.

Type of episode	Treatment
Manic	Review current medications for precipitants and current treatment If on current anti-manic medication, check levels (lithium), and review doses Otherwise, an antipsychotic is usually the first-line treatment. Lithium or valproate should be considered if previous good response (although lithium is less effective for severe symptoms) Both antipsychotics and anti-manic medication may be required
Depressive	If on current medication review the dose, consider a second agent (e.g. lamotrigine) If antidepressant use is warranted, an SSRI, plus an anti-manic drug, is recommended. Quetiapine may also be considered Antidepressant use requires caution in case of a 'switch' to hypomania or mania; also, a positive response may be slow or poor If the antidepressants is ineffective, further options include increasing the dose, switching to an alternative type or adding an antipsychotic or lithium Antidepressants should be stopped 8 weeks after recovery from depression
SSRI, selective serotonin reuptake inhibitor.	

Table 4.4 Pharmacological treatment in acute episodes of bipolar disorder

Precautions that the patient can take include:
- establishing a routine
- ensuring good levels of sleep
- limiting stressors
- avoiding substance abuse
- remaining compliant with treatment regimes

CBT may be useful both for depressive episodes and for addressing false cognitions in mania.

Social

Support with factors such as education, employment and family issues should be offered when required.

Complications/prognosis

The risk of a worse prognosis is increased by:

- early onset
- lower socioeconomic status
- poor social support
- ongoing psychosocial stressors
- longer periods of depression
- psychosis
- frequent relapses
- substance misuse

There is a risk of depression after the successful treatment of mania, in part because of removal of the 'manic defence' against reality. This risk is highest in older people.

Morbidity and mortality

The suicide rate in bipolar disorder is high – approaching 20%. The risk is highest in:

- depressive episodes
- type II illness
- men
- earlier stages of the illness

Patients are also at risk of:

- damage to their reputation, employment and relationships from reckless behaviour
- sexual exploitation, unplanned pregnancy, sexually transmitted infections because of sexual disinhibition and elevated libido
- financial difficulties owing to excessive spending or financial exploitation
- accidental injuries
- self-neglect
- exhaustion due to mania
- substance misuse

4.4 Perinatal psychiatric conditions

Psychiatric disorders associated with birth (**Table 4.5**) range in severity from:

	Maternity blues	**Postnatal depression**	**Puerperal psychosis**
Onset	3–7 days post partum	Usually within 4 weeks post partum	Within 2 weeks post partum
Frequency	66% More common in primiparous patients	10–15% Risk increased by previous depression, marital strife, poor social support, younger age	0.1–0.2% Risk increased by personal/family history of puerperal psychosis or bipolar disorder, puerperal infection, obstetric complications
Symptoms	Tearful Irritability Labile mood Poor sleep	Depression Irritability Labile mood Anxiety Possibly feelings of guilt or failure regarding mothering ability Thoughts of harm to self or baby	Psychosis usually affective (depressive or manic); alternatively delirium (organic) or schizophreniform High risk of suicide and harm to baby
Management	Explanation and reassurance	Supportive explanation and reassurance CBT, IPT Antidepressants Hospital if severe	Exclude organic cause, admission Benzodiazepines/antipsychotics/mood stabilisers/antidepressants/ECT
Prognosis	Usually self-limiting Can lead to postnatal depression if severe	Most improve within 1 month Timely recovery important for child's development No increased risk of depression	Most recover within 6–12 weeks One in three risk of recurrence

Table 4.5 Perinatal psychiatric conditions. CBT, cognitive–behavioural therapy; ECT, electroconvulsive therapy; IPT, interpersonal therapy.

- the 'normal' **maternity blues**, associated with changes in sex hormones and psychological stress; to
- **postnatal depression**, related to factors such as alterations in hormones, a reaction to the significant life-changing events, problems coping and loss of sleep; to
- the most serious – **puerperal psychosis** – in which symptoms such as command hallucinations and delusions of an evil baby can pose high risks

If required, admission is to a mother and baby unit to ensure that bonding is not compromised.

5.1 Clinical scenario

Paracetamol overdose

Presentation

It is 5.30 a.m. and Naomi is referred to the on-call psychiatric senior house officer (SHO). She is a 19 year old originally from south Wales. She has taken an overdose of paracetamol and needs psychiatric assessment.

Diagnostic approach

More information is needed:

- most importantly, has she been attended to fully from a medical point of view? Are the results of blood tests and other investigations known? Until this is the case, there is usually little function in seeing someone.
- has she consumed anything that may impair assessment? This may mean alcohol, recreational drugs or prescription drugs which cause sedation.
- is there any previous psychiatric history? Old medical notes should be obtained and may highlight background factors to her presentation.

Initial history

On admission, Naomi stated she had drunk two bottles of wine in the afternoon before taking the overdose. Her boyfriend and mother are with her and disclose a previous overdose two years ago. Her blood tests have shown no liver damage and low levels of paracetamol at four hours. She will require no further medical treatment in the emergency department.

After finding a private room to talk in, she tells the psychiatry SHO that she took the overdose because she is 'depressed' but regrets it now. She thinks her boyfriend may have cheated on her and, when drunk after an argument the previous day, she took 10 paracetamol. She texted her boyfriend to tell him it was his fault but wrote no suicide note.

Throughout the interview, she maintains good eye contact and is keen to tell the psychiatric SHO everything. Her phone keeps receiving messages from friends asking if everything is alright. She leaves the room briefly to answer a call.

Diagnostic approach

There are five main areas to cover in self-harm assessment:

1. What was the person's **intention** when they harmed themselves? For example, a cry for help, desire to die, not knowing what else to do.
2. Is there **ongoing intent** to die? Is there regret?
3. What are the person's current/likely future **problems**? For example, relationships, finances, physical health.
4. Is there a **psychiatric disorder** present?
5. What **resources** does the patient have? For example, family, friends, GP, counselling.

This (apparently) limited information establishes:

- the intentions she had
- that she regrets her actions
- some of her current problems
- that a wide range of people are supporting her

It seems unlikely that she will have any psychiatric disorder but further screening questions will be useful.

Further history

With Naomi's agreement her mother joins the assessment. She says that binge drinking is an issue and that Naomi's relationships tend to be volatile. She describes Naomi as having been in a good mood the day before when they went shopping together, laughing and joking. They have already decided that Naomi will stay with her mother for a few days, that she will try to cut down on the drinking and that she plans to see the GP about her pill next week anyway.

Diagnostic approach

Assessment following self-harm is daunting, not least because people it is perceived as a long process. However, thorough assessment need not be an endless task. There is nothing to indicate an axis 1 mental illness in this case, but equally there should be no pressure to place a diagnostic label on this event. Simply finding out what happened, observing the aftermath and obtaining a collateral history will give an indication of suicide risk. In this instance, it can be deemed low. Follow-up will be with the GP, and a brief letter outlining the formulation of the assessment should be sent as soon as possible

5.2 Suicide and self-harm

People with persistent thoughts of suicide or those who have presented to medical services following acts of self-harm constitute a large

> All healthy men have thought of their own suicide.
>
> Albert Camus

and important proportion of a psychiatrist's workload.

Following suicide, the classical method of investigating the individual's characteristics is through psychological autopsy. This involves interviewing key informants and reviewing medical records, and has shown psychiatric disorders to be present in over 90% of people who kill themselves.

| Highly lethal, more 'traditional' methods of self-harm often used in suicide | • Hanging, shooting, jumping off a high bridge/building
• Poisoning via herbicides/carbon monoxide
• Stabbing, electrocution, drowning
• Overdose of prescribed or recreational drugs
• Cutting/burning
• Self-biting, scratching, gouging
• Sticking needles into skin
• Interfering with wound healing
• Self-battery, hair pulling
• Exercising to inflict pain |
| Usually less lethal, self-harming methods | • Restricting necessities of life
• Stopping medication
• Deliberate recklessness e.g. when driving |

Figure 5.1 Common methods of suicide and self-harm

Self-harm comprises a wide range of behaviours (**Figure 5.1**), and those who self-harm are a heterogeneous group. More than any other presentation, it arouses ambivalent feelings in healthcare professionals more used to dealing with illness and disease beyond a patient's direct control.

Terminology

Self-harm is a behaviour not an illness. It is an umbrella term for any non-fatal act that has the intent of harming oneself physically. Using the adjective 'deliberate' is now generally avoided because of derogatory connotations. The term 'parasuicide' is sometimes used synonymously with self-harm.

> ### Guiding principle
>
> In many countries, particularly in the Middle East, suicide is a criminal offence. It used to be an offence under English common law but ceased to be so with the passing of the Suicide Act 1961, which also makes it an offence to assist in a suicide.

'**Attempted suicide**' may still be used to distinguish episodes when there is at least some evidence of intent to die.

Suicide is the act of intentionally killing oneself.

Epidemiology

Suicide

Globally, suicide accounts for approximately one million deaths per year, i.e. 1.5% of all deaths. This makes suicide the tenth leading cause of death worldwide, responsible for one death every 40 seconds. Unsurprisingly, the World Health Organization wants to promote suicide prevention strategies in all countries.

These figures are probably an underestimation of the true burden given differences in methods of death recording. For example, in Luxembourg a suicide note is mandatory for demonstrating true intent.

Substantial differences in suicide rates exist between different countries (**Figure 5.2**). In Europe, the rate is generally higher in northern countries (Lithuania, Latvia, Finland) than in southern (Greece, Spain, Portugal). Former Soviet states in particular have very high rates of suicide, and 30% of worldwide suicides occur in China, where it accounts for 3.6% of all

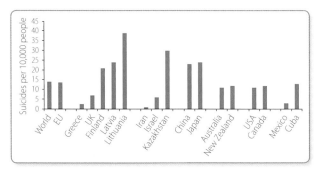

Figure 5.2 Suicide rates around the world

deaths. In the UK, suicide accounts for around 6000 deaths per year, with the highest rate among 15- to 44-year-old men.

The suicide rate peaks in spring, which is perhaps counterintuitive. One theory for this is that the observed 'rebirth' accentuates feelings of hopelessness.

Self-harm

Although self-harm in the form of cutting is described in ancient texts, overdosing is a relatively new phenomenon. Observational studies from the 1960s raised fears of an emerging epidemic and led to cohort studies that confirmed increasing rates of self-harm in successive birth cohorts. Presently, the incidence appears to be stabilising.

The true extent of self-harm is difficult to establish as many may not report the incident or may present to non-medical services, such as the Samaritans in the UK. Between 5% and 9% of Australian, US and English adolescents report self-harming in the previous year. In the UK, there are approximately 170,000 cases seen in hospital per year. Self-poisoning is the most common method requiring admission to hospital, followed by self-injury, usually in the form of cutting.

The male–female ratio is 1:1.3. Self-harm is much more common in younger age groups, is usually impulsive and is frequently accompanied by alcohol and drug abuse.

Causes/pathogenesis

Suicide

Table 5.1 outlines the aetiological and risk factors in suicide.

Suicide prevention   The UK National Confidential Inquiry into Suicide and Homicide (2001) found that one-quarter of people who went on to commit suicide had contact with mental health services in the year preceding the event; 22% of these were perceived as having been preventable.

All medical professionals, and GPs in particular, need to be alert to the patient seeking help. Sixty per cent of those committing suicide consult a GP in the six months before the event, and 40% within weeks. It is estimated that two-thirds of those committing suicide disclose their intention to someone beforehand. The inpatient suicide rate is highest in the first week of admission, usually by hanging, and there is a spike in suicide risk following discharge from hospital.

Prevention strategies have been set up in many countries. The focus is essentially divided into:

- targeting high-risk groups: e.g. screening depressed patients for suicidal ideation and, if present, proceeding to detailed risk assessment
- population-based strategies: these aim to remove the access to means, provide social support and reduce stress (e.g. reducing unemployment); recent successful examples include the change from toxic coal gas to non-toxic North Sea gas in the 1960s, the introduction of catalytic convertors to cars and the reduction in paracetamol pack sizes

Self-harm

The aetiological factors for self-harm vary widely, although they are similar to those for completed suicide. Common reasons

> **Clinical insight**
>
> Remember also to consider individuals' protective factors. Religious belief, for example, is correlated with reduced self-harm and suicide. This should include their personal 'reasons' to live, e.g. children, friends and work.
>
> The suicide rate in depression is approximately 4%; in bipolar disorder 10–15%; and in schizophrenia 4–5%.

Biological	Psychological	Social
Predisposing		
Previous suicide attempt: lifetime risk 10–15%	Sexual abuse	Low socioeconomic status
Previous self-harm: lifetime risk 3–5%	Childhood adversity	Living alone
Sex: males 3–4 times higher rate of suicide. Probably due to choice of more violent means	Impulsive personality traits	Single, widowed, separated or divorced
	Low self-esteem	Unemployment
Age: highest in 25–44 age group		Country of residence
History of mental illness or substance misuse		Occupation: stressful jobs with access to lethal means → higher rates of suicide, e.g. doctors, vets, farmers
Family history of self-harm or mental illness		
Precipitating		
Chronic/debilitating physical illness (e.g. cancer, epilepsy, multiple sclerosis)	Life stressors, particularly bereavement or criminal invovlement	Availability of means (drugs, firearms, pesticides)
Painful physical illness → particularly vulnerable	Hopelessness	Lethality of means
Initial recovery period from severe depression as energy and motivation levels increase but suicidal ideas persist; may account for observed increase in suicidality after initiation of pharmacotherapy	Discharge following psychiatric hospitalisation (highest rate in the first 1–2 weeks following discharge)	Media contagion effect: clustering of suicidal acts is not uncommon
Recent diagnosis of schizophrenia		Economic recession
Delusions of control, poverty or guilt	Missed last clinic appointment	Natural disasters
Intoxication		
Maintaining	–	–
Untreated/undertreated mental illness		
Non-compliance with medication		

Table 5.1 Aetiology and risk factors for suicide

Clinical insight

Triggers of self-harm and suicide: adverse life events, such as interpersonal conflict or relationship breakdown, are well known to 'trigger' self-harm. When Diana, Princess of Wales, was killed in 1997 there was an increased rate of self-harm in the following week. Clustering of self-harm and suicide has occasionally been described, especially in younger people. In the late 2000s, a spate of suicides occurred in the Bridgend area of South Wales. This 'contagion effect' probably results from sensationalist media reporting and, more controversially, internet social networking sites.

are a cry for help, a reflection of poor coping strategies, impulsive personality traits, a failed suicide attempt, self-punishment and substituting psychological distress for physical pain.

Clinical features

Table 5.2 compares the characteristics of those with completed suicide against non-fatal deliberate self-harm.

Understanding self-harm is impossible without consideration of intent. Although lethality and suicidal intent are strongly correlated, one recent study showed only two out of three survivors of near-fatal self-harm had suicidal thoughts. Most people admitted to hospital following an overdose neither want nor expect to die, and although self-harm (particularly near-fatal self-harm) is a major risk factor for suicide, most survivors are still alive at five years.

Approach to the patient

The overall aim following an act of self-harm (or when a patient expresses suicidal ideation) is assessing the likelihood of suicidal ideas progressing to acts. This is an opportunity for thorough assessment and for a therapeutic consultation in which the problems leading to the act can be addressed. It is important not to be punitive as this will discourage a patient from seeking help in the future.

Investigations and management

Following any act of self-harm, the following should be carried out:
- medical treatment
- full psychiatric history
- risk assessment

	Non-fatal self-harm	Completed suicide
Sex	Female > male	Male > female
Age	Adolescence/early 20s	Middle age onwards
Marital status	Single	Widowed > divorced > single > married
Social class	IV and V Unemployed	I and V Unemployed and retired
Childhood events	Broken home, unstructured	Death of parent
Family history	Self-harm	Depression, substance misuse, suicide
Physical health	Usually healthy	Prominent physical health problems
Personality	Antisocial, borderline, histrionic personality traits	–
Season	All	Spring (April–June)
Diagnosis	'Mental distress' Personality disorder 'Reactive' depression	Depression: 70% Alcoholism: 15% Schizophrenia
Precipitants	Situational crisis	Guilt Hopelessness
Method and context	Overdose and cutting Impulsive Others present Prior/early disclosure of actions	Violent methods Planned Alone Precautions against discovery Suicide note

Table 5.2 Contrasting profiles of typical completed suicide and non-fatal self-harm

- immediate management
- follow-up

Medical treatment

This may include a toxicology screen, blood tests, assessment of alcohol levels, suturing, etc. If a patient declines treatment, their capacity to do so must be assessed. Treatment depends on the method of self-harm, but can include antidotes, e.g. N-acetyl cysteine for paracetamol overdose or naloxone for opiate overdose. Consult the appropriate national database if uncertain; in the UK this is TOXBASE (the primary clinical toxicology database of the National Poisons Information Service), found at http://www.toxbase.org/.

A patient must be physically stable before conducting psychiatric assessment. In particular, assessment of a drowsy or intoxicated patient is unlikely to be reliable.

Full psychiatric history

A full psychiatric history is required to establish what happened. Remember that the act of listening to someone's problems sympathetically can be therapeutic in itself, and establishing a good rapport is crucial.

The assessment should encompass:

- the story of exactly what happened; this should include enquiry about intent to die
- consideration of aetiological factors and factors protecting against suicide (**Tables 5.1** and **5.3**)
- consideration of possible comorbid acute and chronic psychiatric diagnoses
- assessment of the social circumstances (i.e. living environment, support network, etc.)
- attitude towards the future (i.e. desire to be 'alive', desire to receive help, and hopelessness)
- if possible, a collateral history

Risk assessment

This may include (judicious) use of tools such as the SAD PERSONS Scale. Remember that checklists cannot replace clinical judgement, and access to means should also be considered.

Immediate interventions

Discuss the case with a senior member of staff/colleague and formulate a management plan. Aim to decrease the short-term

Indicators of serious suicidal intent	Indicators of lower risk
Planned and premeditated	Impulsive attempt with/without influence of alcohol
Carried out in isolation with precautions taken against discovery	Attempt performed in front of others
Final acts in anticipation of death, e.g. paying all bills and writing a suicide note	No preparatory acts
Violent methods (e.g. hanging/shooting)	Non-violent method (e.g. overdose)
Belief that the act would be final and irreversible	Uncertainty about the outcome
Not seeking help afterwards	Help sought or people alerted after the act
Regret or ambivalence about surviving	Relief at being alive

Table 5.3 Indicators of higher and lower suicidal risk

risk of repetition and completed suicide, and consider the following in turn.

Refer or not refer? Most cases of self-harm require no ongoing specialist input and patients can be discharged to the care of the GP or community mental health team (CMHT) with clear and prompt communication. If there is concern, mental illness or if the individual is under 18, a psychiatric opinion should generally be sought.

Admit or not admit? All under 16s presenting outside working hours be admitted overnight to a paediatric ward for next day assessment. In adults, only a small proportion of patients will be admitted to psychiatric hospital (approximately 3%). Admission may be under mental health legislation if necessary, although, in practice, structures such as crisis teams are often used to avoid admission.

A shared understanding Try to reach a shared understanding of the meaning of the behaviour and identify the patient's needs. A plan should be made for what the patient would do if they felt like this again, including who they would tell and how they would get help.

Provide practical help with precipitating factors This may be as simple as discussing solutions to a particular problem faced by the patient or include referral or signposting to social services, counselling, substance addiction services, etc.

Practical advice to allay fears Simple advice to give people with thoughts of suicide or self-harm includes:
- reminding them that they have not always felt this way and will not always feel this way
- reminding them that the risk of committing suicide is highest in the combined presence of (1) suicidal thoughts, (2) the means to commit suicide and (3) the opportunity to commit suicide; therefore, if the patient is prone to suicidal thoughts tell them not to be alone and to try to remove any means, e.g. giving tablets/knives to a friend or relative
- reminding them to share problems, ideally with a friend or relative or, alternatively, with organisations such as the Samaritans, their GP or an emergency department; this promotes adaptive expression of emotions
- advising them to avoid alcohol or drugs as these can increase impulsive behaviour
- recommending that they get some good sleep as this can significantly change one's outlook
- distracting themselves; this can include speaking with someone, watching television, writing, drawing, playing a musical instrument or exercising
- trying relaxation techniques such as deep breathing or yoga to reduce tension
- if they are unable to resist self-harm, to try squeezing ice cubes, fitting rubber bands around their wrist or biting something strongly flavoured, e.g. a lemon or a chilli
- avoiding unmonitored online forums

- making a list of positive things about themselves and their life; and keeping this and reading it when plagued by thoughts of self-harm
- writing a safety plan (when well) and discussing it with their GP, psychiatrist or community psychiatric nurse

Communicate your assessment Lastly, communicate your agreed assessment and follow-up plans with the patient and their GP. With the patient's consent, their family should also be informed of the results of the assessment and their support mobilised. The patient's family can be an invaluable tool to ongoing monitoring of mental state.

Follow-up interventions

A clear follow-up plan should be made before discharge. There is little point in making a follow-up appointment if the patient does not want to engage. Ideally, they should be provided with written information about services appropriate to them.

Follow-up can include:
- review with their GP or CMHT
- a one-off clinic appointment for further assessment
- referral to specialist services for treatment such as counselling, addiction management or brief psychotherapy
- referral for treatment of underlying mental illness, monitoring and support

Prognosis
Self-harm

Self-harm is one of the strongest predictors of future suicide: 20% of people who self-harm repeat the act, and 1% die during the course of the next year. After 9 years, over 5% will have committed suicide. There is a 100-fold increased risk of completed suicide compared with the general population. This means that 10% of people who self-harm eventually complete suicide.

Personality disorders

6.1 Clinical scenario

Concern about a patient in police custody

Presentation

Barry, a 26-year-old man, was arrested for drink-driving by the police. The police officer states that he was extremely aggressive upon arrest, requiring restraint before being taken to police cells. He has a previous history of shoplifting, threatening behaviour, being drunk and disorderly and domestic violence and has had two short custodial sentences. Apparently, he calmed down once taken to the cells and started crying, telling police he is being treated for depression by his GP and had previously been admitted to psychiatric hospital. The police seek a psychiatric assessment as, when left unobserved, he self-harms with a fork.

Diagnostic approach

This information alone strongly indicates a personality disorder of the dissocial or borderline subtype. Multiple, long-standing problems of criminality, alcohol misuse and violence appear prominent. Collateral history and information will be important, as will reviewing previous psychiatric notes. The differential diagnoses to consider are depression, hypomania, psychosis, substance addiction/misuse and malingering. Barry potentially poses a risk to personal safety and should be approached considering this, for example with an officer present and in a safe environment. His mental state should not be assessed until he is sober.

Initial history

Barry appears well kempt, well built and covered in tattoos. He is extremely nonchalant given the gravity of the

> ## Clinical insight
>
> **Malingering** is the intentional falsification of symptoms of illness for a secondary gain, e.g. compensation, obtaining prescriptions or, as in Clinical scenario 6.1, avoiding criminal charges.

charges, shows disregard for authority and a complete lack of remorse. He blames all his actions on his 'depression'. Exploring this, it becomes apparent that his wife recently threw him out for cheating and he thinks he has been 'depressed' for the past five days. There are no features to indicate hypomania and he binge drinks but is not dependent on alcohol.

His notes state that he is the fifth of eight siblings and had a violent alcoholic father. A child psychiatrist diagnosed him with conduct disorder.

The cuts on his forearm are relatively superficial but require cleaning and bandaging.

Diagnostic approach

This information supports a diagnosis of personality disorder. The aetiological factors in his behavioural pattern might be the family history of criminality, childhood physical and emotional abuse, probable parental discord and childhood conduct disorder. The precipitating factors for recent events appear to be the breakdown of his relationship, and the self-harm appears to have been precipitated by contact with the police.

Further history

With Barry's permission, a collateral history from his estranged wife is obtained. She is still angry with him. He has had multiple affairs. Their relationship was volatile and she describes him as 'having a short fuse'. She says that he always blames his problems with the police on someone or something else but never seems to learn from the experience. She has no concerns about any symptoms of depression.

Diagnostic approach

Given the collateral history, personality disorder can be diagnosed. There is a high level of personal distress and social disruption and the patient meets many criteria for dissocial personality disorder (**Table 6.1**).

Management in this situation is challenging, and psychiatric services may have only a limited role to play. The diagnosis should be explained to the police and it should be clarified whether they intend to proceed with charges. They may be

Cluster	DSM IV	ICD-10	Characteristics	Differential diagnoses
A	Paranoid	Paranoid	Sensitive to setbacks Bears grudges Suspiciousness of others Combative/tenacious sense of personal rights Possessive/jealous of partners Excessive self-importance Belief in conspiracy theories	Schizophrenia Persistent delusional disorder
	Schizoid	Schizoid	Excessive introspection and fantasy Lack of close relationships Solitary activities Insensitivity to social norms Emotionally cold Apparent indifference to praise or criticism Anhedonia Disinterest in sexual partners	Asperger's syndrome Schizophrenia Agoraphobia Social phobia Depression
	Schizotypal	N/A (classified with schizophrenia and related disorders)	Oddities of appearance, behaviour, speech and thinking, similar to those seen in schizophrenia Fear of social interaction High probability of 'conversion' to schizophrenia	Schizophrenia and related disorders

Table 6.1a   Cluster A personality disorders: types, features and common differential diagnoses

Cluster	DSM IV	ICD-10	Characteristics	Differential diagnoses
B	Antisocial	Dissocial	Callous lack of concern for others Irresponsibility, irritability and aggression Irritability and aggression Fiery, turbulent, short-lived relationships Blaming of others History of conduct disorder in childhood	Psychotic episode Substance misuse
B	Borderline	Emotionally unstable (subcategorised into impulsive* OR borderline)	Unstable affect and explosive behaviour Impulsivity and inability to plan Multiple turbulent relationships Recurrent emotional 'crises' Stress-related psychotic symptoms Unclear self-image Sensitivity to criticism Fear of abandonment Suicide attempts and self-harm	Depression Bipolar disorder Adjustment disorder Psychosis Adult attention deficit and hyperactivity disorder (ADHD)
B	Histrionic	Histrionic	Self-dramatisation Theatricality Exaggerated expression of emotions Persistently manipulative Suggestible	Hypomania/mania Substance misuse
B	Narcissistic	(–)	Grandiosity Lack of empathy Hypersensitivity to evaluation by others	

Table 6.1b Cluster B personality disorders: types, features and common differential diagnoses

Cluster	DSM IV	ICD-10	Characteristics	Differential diagnoses
C	Avoidant	Anxious (avoidant)	Avoids social contact Preoccupation with being criticised or rejected in social situations Yearning to be liked and accepted Restricted lifestyle Persistent feelings of tension Apprehensiveness Feelings of ineptitude and inferiority	Social phobia Autistic spectrum disorder
C	Dependent	Dependent	Pervasive reliance on other people Fear of abandonment Weak/inadequate response to the demands of daily life Relinquishing responsibility to others Undue compliance with the wishes of others Excessive need for reassurance	Learning disability Cognitive impairment Anxiety disorder
C	Obsessive–compulsive	Anankastic	Indecisiveness, doubt and excessive caution Perfectionism and excessive attention to detail Adherence to 'rules' Inability to complete tasks Rigidity and stubbornness Exclusion of pleasure and relationships Dominated by intrusive thoughts	Obsessive–compulsive disorder Autistic spectrum disorder

* Impulsive type (ICD-10) appears to be a crossover between dissocial and borderline having characteristics of both

Table 6.1c Cluster C personality disorders: types, features and common differential diagnoses

reluctant to do so in view of the possible psychiatric condition. The police should be assured that if he is to be kept in custody, further psychiatric input can be arranged.

A thorough risk assessment is very important here. Admission in this case would not be indicated; however, sometimes short-term admission for further observation and during crises is helpful, especially if there is diagnostic uncertainty. There is no role for medication. Engagement with psychological treatments is indicated, but often proves difficult in such cases. Finally, it should not be assumed that if a patient is diagnosed with personality disorder, they may not also have an acute mental illness in the future.

6.2 Personality disorders

Personality refers to the characteristic behaviours, emotions and cognitive attributes of a person. In this manner, we may identify the 'happy-go-lucky postman', the 'anxious and pernickety schoolmistress', the 'charming and confident salesman' and so on.

An individual's personality consists of certain characteristics, which are referred to as traits.

Personality traits are defined in DSM-IV as 'enduring patterns of perceiving, relating to, and thinking about the environment and oneself … exhibited in a wide range of important social and personal contexts'. Personality traits become apparent by mid-adolescence; they generally remain stable into adulthood, but can be accentuated by stress. In some individuals, certain personality traits may become extreme, inflexible and maladaptive, and so cause problems to the person or society. This is termed personality disorder.

The history of personality disorder is complex but fascinating. Terminology, as in many other psychiatric disorders, has changed many times, there have been a multitude of different aetiological theories and, as an area, it has generated great deal of controversy (**Section 6.3**).

Clinical insight

The term 'borderline' originates from the idea that borderline disorder lay somewhere between the older notions of neurosis and psychosis.

Epidemiology

Community rates of personality disorder are estimated to be 10%. This figure subsumes all the different categories of personality disorder. Antisocial personality disorder has a prevalence of 2%; borderline 1.5%; and schizoid 0.5%.

In primary care, 5–8% of people being treated for 'psychiatric conditions' will have a primary diagnosis of personality disorder, whereas 20–30% will have comorbid personality disorder. It is associated with a greater frequency of consultation and increased use of psychotropic medication.

In secondary care, 30–40% of psychiatric outpatients and 40–60% of inpatients will have a diagnosis of personality disorder, but not usually as the primary diagnosis. In prison populations, the prevalence of personality disorder can be as high as 78%, usually categorised as antisocial or borderline.

Overall, there is an excess of personality disorder in younger adults and urban communities. Prevalence is approximately equal for men and women; however, certain subtypes are diagnosed more often depending on sex (e.g. antisocial personality disorder in men and borderline/histrionic personality disorder in women).

Causes

The exact cause of personality disorders is unknown; however, countless theories have been proposed. Personality disorder as an attenuated form of axis 1 disorders is certainly worthy of consideration. Cluster A disorders have much in common with schizophrenic spectrum disorders whereas cluster C disorders share symptomatology with the **neurotic**, **stress-related** and **somatoform** disorders.

Genetic and environmental factors probably contribute in equal measure to personality.

Genetics

There is evidence for a moderate genetic contribution to personality traits (e.g. 35–50% heritability for neuroticism and extraversion). A family history of personality disorder, depression and alcohol dependency also predisposes to the disorder.

Temperament refers to the aspects of personality that are thought to be innate rather than learned. In childhood, factors such as irritability, activity, attention span, frequency of smiling and approach to unfamiliar people or events are typically considered. Childhood temperament, even at 3 years old, has been found to predict personality and personality disorders in adulthood.

Environmental and experiential factors

Psychological theories of personality disorders generally relate adverse early life experiences and problems with early attachment to later difficulties in emotional development and interpersonal relationships. A disruptive early environment filled with trauma, neglect and chaos may lead to defensive, maladaptive personality patterns in vulnerable individuals. This may reflect social learning (i.e. copying the behaviour of, say, a violent parent). It is not known why most people who experience traumatic childhoods are resilient and lead normal lives whereas in others it seems to precipitate mental illness or personality disorder.

Clinical features

Personality disorders are unified by the following features:

- there is a deeply ingrained and enduring pattern of inner experience and behaviour which manifests as **inflexible responses** to a range of social situations
- the behaviour **deviates markedly** from the prevailing cultural norms
- they are evident in **multiple domains** of behaviour and psychological functioning – cognition, affect, impulse control and interpersonal relationships
- the person experiences subjective **distress and impairment** in social functioning
- the **onset** is evident in childhood or adolescence

After these criteria are met, diagnosis requires the presence of certain specific and distinct features. This so-called 'categorical' approach is used in both ICD-10 and DSM-IV. ICD-10 divides personality disorders into eight types, although the validity and reliability of these is unclear. Often, patients fit into several categories either fully or partially, or do not fit well into any.

DSM-IV groups similar types of disorder using three clusters (A, B and C), each of which encompasses several categories (**Tables 6.1a-6.1c**). Cluster A includes individuals with personality disorders classified as 'odd or eccentric'; cluster B includes those who are 'dramatic, emotional or erratic'; and cluster C includes those who are 'anxious or fearful'.

The specific features of each personality disorder are given in **Tables 6.1a-6.1c**.

Common presentations of personality disorder

People with cluster A and C disorders are less likely to come to the attention of medical professionals. The common presenting complaints of individuals with personality disorder are:

- deliberate self-harm
- aggression and violence
- anxiety and depression
- alcohol and substance misuse

Clinical insight

A patient's current mental state, recent life events, substance use and a multitude of other factors can influence the history given. It is unlikely that a diagnosis of personality disorder can (or should) be made at a first clinical meeting.

Approach to the patient

A thorough history and mental state examination are essential. Particular emphasis should be paid to the following:

- **past psychiatric history**: contact with mental health services, nature of that contact, self-harm, detailed history of admissions
- **drug history**: medication used and success thereof, substance misuse
- **developmental history**: perinatal trauma, developmental milestones
- **family history**: family dynamics, family history of psychiatric illness, substance misuse, criminality, parents' personalities
- **personal history**: detailed account of childhood and adolescence, schooling, truancy and other delinquent behaviour,

occupational history (frequent job changes?), psychosexual history, history of physical or sexual abuse, forensic history, concept of self, coping strategies, gambling; aim to establish whether there are recurring patterns of behaviour or emotional response and their impact

- **collateral history**: this is essential for a valid diagnosis and should be obtained from as many sources as feasible
- **Mental state examination**: there may be subjective low mood, transient psychotic symptoms, ideas of reference, evidence of self-harm

Micropsychotic episodes

Persistent psychotic symptoms such as delusions, hallucinations or formal thought disorder are not a feature of personality disorder. However, transient psychotic experiences ('micropsychotic episodes') can occur. Compared with true schizophreniform psychoses, they are more short-lived and directly related to a given (usually stressful/unpleasant) situation. Medication or hospitalisation are not required as a rule.

Personality assessment

Assess:

- **relationships**: assess quality and quantity of intimate relationships, friendships, attitude to work colleagues, superiors and those in authority
- **predominant mood**: irritable, anger management issues, despondent, fluctuating, how feelings are shown
- **character**: shy/self-conscious, outgoing, impulsive, self-esteem, rigidity, tidiness
- **leisure activities**

Clinical insight

If you suspect a personality disorder, it is often useful to make a list of 'abnormal' personality traits and describe the impact of these on occupation, family life, relationships and other domains.

Investigations

It is important to differentiate personality change from personality disorder. If there is an indication of personality change, an organic aetiology is possible, requiring physical examination and neuroimaging.

Investigations should include further interview(s), including collateral history.

Personality questionnaires such as the Minnesota Multi-phasic Personality Inventory (MMPI), Personality Assessment Schedule (PAS), Cattell's 16 Personality Factor Questionnaire (16PF) and the Eynsenck Personality Questionnaire can provide further detailed evaluation of personality.

Diagnostic criteria and differential diagnoses

Tables 6.1a-6.1c show the personality disorder categories identified by DSM-IV and ICD-10. A patient must satisfy general criteria for a personality disorder **and** a certain number of listed features. It is not uncommon for individuals to meet criteria for more than one category. All categories for which a person meets criteria should be considered as, clinically, it is more important to describe and understand an individual's problems than pigeonhole them into an ill-fitting group. If they meet criteria for two or more groups, they do not have more than one disorder as a person has one personality.

Specific differential diagnoses are given in **Table 6.1**. Remember that personality disorders are classified as axis II disorders (in DSM-IV) and the presence of personality disorder does not preclude a comorbid axis I disorder such as depression.

Management

Personality disorders are treatable, but these patients are often highly time-consuming and can engender negative feelings in professionals because of the nature of their presentation (threats, abuse, forensic records, crises and general 'noise').

General principles

The general principles of management are:

- to be realistic about goals and available resources
- to identify an individual able to form a stable, long-term therapeutic relationship
- that multidisciplinary and agency work is usually required

- that structure, consistency and clear boundaries (e.g. acceptable and unacceptable behaviours) must be a foundation of treatment to promote responsibility for the patient's own actions
- to use a care programme approach (CPA) or contract to plan for 'crises'. CPAs are written agreed long-term care plans headed by an allocated co-ordinator. They are reviewed regularly in order to meet the evolving needs of the patient
- that inpatient treatment is rarely indicated even at times of crisis. Admission can be adverse as it may accentuate feelings of abandonment and reinforce the behaviour; however, it may reduce the short-term risk of suicide or enable assessment of comorbid illness.
- to treat any underlying or comorbid psychiatric disorders; the diagnosis of personality disorder should not prevent consideration of comorbidity
- to identify and reinforce skills and positive traits, thereby helping to find a lifestyle which suits the patient and maximises their potential, e.g. a job with a high requirement for perfectionism but in an understanding environment in someone with anankastic personality disorder
- to treat or address specific behavioural and social problems, e.g. anger, self-harm, self-esteem, housing or finance problems
- that risk assessment is very important given the substantial suicide rate and risks posed to others

Clinical insight

Short admission on a voluntary basis is preferable to long periods of 'assessment' under the terms of mental health legislation such as the Mental Health Act in England and Wales.

Medication

Generally, medication should be used as an adjunct to psychosocial treatments; always keep in mind *primum non nocere* ('first do no harm'). Medication is used on a 'trial' basis to treat symptoms rather than the disorder. Target symptoms need to be identified (e.g. aggression, impulsivity, depressive symptoms) and there should be discussion of the risk–benefit profile. The simplest regimen possible should be prescribed for a limited time period, and the success or otherwise reviewed on a regular basis.

Low-dose antipsychotics There is some evidence that low-dose antipsychotics reduce impulsivity, self-harm and aggression. Fluoxetine may have a similar effect.

Antidepressants Their use has had only equivocal success in treating depressive symptoms; toxicity in overdose should always be considered.

Mood stabilisers These include lithium, carbamazepine and sodium valproate and can also reduce aggression and mood fluctuations, but tolerability and toxicity are more of a problem.

Psychotherapy
Co-operation is a prerequisite. A broad range of approaches mainly using ideas from cognitive–behavioural therapy and psychoanalysis have been used. Dialectical–behavioural therapy has been shown to be effective in decreasing self-harm rates, and cognitive analytical therapy has also been used with some success.

Therapeutic communities
A daily programme of group or individual therapy, social and cultural events and educational or work placements should be organised. The fundamental idea is that, by forming relationships in a positive, trusting environment where one is valued, accepted and supported, the cycle of maladaptive behaviour can be broken. Community members set rules and manage the group (together with skilled staff) and participate in groups that share and confront problems as they arise.

Outcomes are variable, but those who manage to commit to the group use less medication and have fewer admissions to hospital.

Complications/prognosis

Classically, personality was seen as 'untreatable', although there is mounting evidence to indicate that this is not the case. Outcomes do, however, vary widely. As patients get older, behavioural symptoms may improve, whereas cognitive and affective symptoms remain. As a general guide, of the DSM-IV clusters:

A Worsens with age
B Improves with age: there is less aggression but relationships remain poor. In borderline personality disorder, 50% no longer meet the diagnostic threshold at 10- to 25-year follow-up. Within the same cluster, however, dissocial personality disorder does poorly
C Stays the same

The main complications of personality disorders include:

- disruption to relationships, education and employment (and society)
- a possible **predisposition** to psychiatric disorders, especially alcohol and substance misuse and depression
- possible **coexistence** with other psychiatric disorders, which can worsen the prognosis of both disorders
- that they may be **mistaken for** psychiatric disorders and thereby inappropriately treated
- perpetuation of a cycle of child abuse and domestic violence
- subjective distress
- a high incidence of deliberate self-harm (60–80% in cluster B) and suicide (9% in cluster B). This is a similar mortality to that for psychosis; 30–60% of those who complete suicide have evidence of personality disorder
- violence and other criminal activities

6.3 Controversies in the field of personality disorders

Illness and stigma

In an area characterised by disagreement, it is surprising that most psychiatrists agree that personality disorder is not a 'mental illness'. Some argue therefore that, if it is not an illness, why medicalise personality? One man's 'disorder' is another man's virtue: e.g. perfectionism in anankastic personality disorder. This belief that personality disorder is not an illness has perhaps led to the unhelpful dichotomy between those with illnesses deserving of sympathy, care and treatment and those with personality disorder who tend to be rejected and held responsible for their condition or behaviour. It is not surprising therefore that a diagnosis of personality disorder is sometimes used as justification for therapeutic nihilism

Tautology

This is the circularity of arguing that a patient displays clinical features suggestive of the disorder, which are then explained by the fact that they have that disorder. For example, a patient may have recurrent impulsive acts of self-harm following minor setbacks and be diagnosed with borderline personality disorder. It is then rather self-serving to say that they impulsively self-harm and are sensitive to setbacks because they have borderline personality disorder

Relationship to other conditions

The relationship between personality and other psychiatric conditions is unclear. Several schools of thought exist, believing that personality disorder cannot occur simultaneously with mental illness, all people with psychiatric illness have personality disorder, some people with personality disorder develop concurrent mental illness, and, finally, that personality disorder is a chronic minor psychosis or neurosis as many symptoms overlap

Unreliability of diagnosis

Personality disorder is one of the more unreliable diagnoses, but once the label is given it tends to remain. Many patients feel that it is a pejorative term applied to difficult people

The antipsychiatry argument

Antipsychiatrists would argue that the personality disorder label (and other diagnoses) is a tool to control undesirable elements in society. For example, in the UK particular controversy surrounded the DSPD (dangerous and severe personality disorder) programme. Launched in 1999, this allowed the indefinite detention and treatment of violent and sexual offenders whom most psychiatrists considered untreatable.

chapter 7

Anxiety disorders and medically unexplained symptoms

This chapter broadly follows the ICD-10 classification of neurotic, stress-related, and somatoform disorders (**Table 7.1**).

> Who's not sat tense before his own heart's curtain.
>
> Rainer Maria Rilke

7.1 Clinical scenario

Ritualistic behaviours

Presentation

Andrew is a 30-year-old man, presenting for the first time to the psychiatric team.

He reports having developed a need to check that his water and gas taps are turned off before he can leave the house or go to bed. This started after his delivery van was held up by armed men a year ago.

Diagnostic approach

Andrew's checking behaviour indicates possible obsessive–compulsive disorder (OCD). This, and the traumatic-sounding hold-up, should be explored further within a full history and Mental State Examination.

History

Andrew describes feeling compelled to stare at the taps, sometimes for an hour, in order to prevent a flood or fire. He knows that this is 'irrational' and it causes him considerable distress.

Group	Key individual disorder
Anxiety disorders	
Phobic anxiety disorders	Agoraphobia Social phobias Specific (isolated) phobias
Other anxiety disorders	Panic disorder Generalised anxiety disorder Mixed anxiety and depressive disorder
Obsessive–compulsive disorder	–
Stress and adjustment disorders	Acute stress reaction Post-traumatic stress disorder Adjustment disorders
Dissociative (conversion) disorders	–
Somatoform disorders	–

Table 7.1 Classification of anxiety disorders and medically unexplained symptoms

The time he needs to stare has increased in the past month, making him late for work.

Other similar symptoms include hesitating for long periods before crossing the road while he struggles to decide whether it is safe to do so.

During the hold-up, Andrew was threatened with a gun, and feared that he would be killed. He declined the counselling offered by his employer, but no longer drives, having switched to a 'stressful' desk job.

Around two months ago he started having nightmares and flashbacks of the hold-up. These have increased gradually in frequency, and he has begun to feel 'constantly on edge … and jumping at all loud noises'.

Asking further about anxiety symptoms reveals that, alongside palpitations and sweating, Andrew occasionally feels as though he is 'in a dream', with 'tunnel vision' in which 'everything is surrounded by an edge'. Sometimes he progresses through a day 'as if on rails, like a train driver'. Investigations of both his heart and his eyes have been unremarkable.

Diagnostic approach

Andrew's description indicates symptoms of both OCD and post-traumatic stress disorder (PTSD). He has various symptoms of anxiety, including derealisation and depersonalisation. It is important to seek any concurrent depression and substance abuse, as these are commonly linked to anxiety disorders.

After the completion of a full assessment, management strategies for this complex case can be considered.

7.2 Anxiety disorders in general

This chapter discusses general aspects of anxiety disorders. Specific anxiety disorders (**Table 7.1**) are discussed in subsequent chapters.

We have all experienced the symptoms of anxiety. A normal response to life events, anxiety is a varied set of physical and psychological symptoms induced by apprehension of a perceived threat. It is a protective mechanism developed through evolution, which affords us the chance of avoiding or escaping potentially dangerous situations.

Anxiety becomes pathological if it is sufficiently excessive in quantity or quality to impair a person's normal functioning.

Epidemiology

Anxiety disorders are common, with a lifetime prevalence of up to 30% in the general population. Prevalence rates for individual conditions are shown in **Table 7.2**.

They tend to begin in early adulthood, although onset can be later in life. Most of these conditions are commoner in women, except social phobia and OCD, which affect both genders equally.

Causes/pathogenesis

The anxiety response

Anxiety is a natural response to a threat and involves the amygdala and hippocampus of the limbic system activating the hypothalamic–pituitary–adrenal (HPA) axis and the sympathetic nervous system. The amygdala helps to process

Anxiety disorder	Prevalence (%)
Generalised anxiety disorder	3.4
Obsessive–compulsive disorder	2.4
Panic disorder	1.6
Specific phobia	8.3
Agoraphobia	4.9
Social phobia	2.0
Post-traumatic stress disorder	3.6
Source: Mental Health: A Report of the Surgeon General 1999.	

Table 7.2 One-year best estimate prevalence rates for adults aged 18–54

threats and fear and has significant connections to parts of the prefrontal (executive) cortex.

Sympathetic nervous system Activation of the sympathetic nervous system, by increased activity of noradrenergic projections from the locus coeruleus in the brainstem, leads to the fight-or-flight response. This prepares the body for immediate action, with physiological changes including a faster heartbeat, increased respiratory rate and heightened attention.

Hypothalamic–pituitary–adrenal axis The HPA axis produces cortisol, via the actions of corticotrophin-releasing hormone and adrenocorticotrophic hormone. Cortisol release initiates widespread adaptive responses to stress. These are useful acutely, but chronically raised levels are damaging, e.g. impairing the immune system and causing hippocampal atrophy.

Anxiety disorders In these disorders there is abnormal or exaggerated arousal. This might be due to a lack of cortical (top-down) control of the limbic system's responses to stimuli, but the exact mechanisms are unclear. Various neurotransmitter imbalances and dysfunction of the HPA axis have been demonstrated in anxiety, but such changes are shared by several psychiatric and medical conditions.

Genetics

There is evidence of a genetic contribution in anxiety disorders, although no specific genes have been identified.

Twin studies demonstrate a genetic predisposition to generalised anxiety disorder (GAD), and both anxiety disorders and 'neurotic' traits (e.g. anxious, obsessional, depressive) appear to run in families.

It has been suggested that there are broad vulnerability periods, including childhood and adolescence, when environmental factors combine with genetic susceptibility to lead to anxiety disorders.

Environmental

Specific childhood factors that can increase the risk of later anxiety include:
- traumatic experiences such as abuse or neglect
- family disruption
- overprotective parents

Throughout life, anxiety disorders can be triggered and perpetuated by stressful life events.

Psychological

Behavioural theories These include:
- classical conditioning (a neutral stimulus begins to elicit a fear response after it is repeatedly associated with a frightening stimulus)
- vicarious learning (adopting the witnessed behaviour of others to a threat)

Cognitive theories These propose that people with anxiety have
- a tendency to think negatively and catastrophise, or
- a perception of being unable to control the environment, leading to feelings of helplessness

Psychodynamic theories These consider that
- anxiety symptoms are secondary to unresolved conflicts, perhaps from childhood development

- the origin of a phobia may be interpreted as the subconscious defence mechanism of displacing fears onto an unrelated situation or object

> ## Clinical insight
>
> - **Depersonalisation** is the sensation that you are no longer in your mind or body, e.g. an 'out of body experience'
> - **Derealisation** is the sensation that the world around you is not real
>
> Both can be caused by anxiety, temporal lobe epilepsy, depression and fatigue/sleep deprivation.

Comorbidities

Anxiety is associated with various other conditions, such as those in **Table 7.3**.

Clinical features

The symptoms of anxiety can be separated into psychological and somatic/physical categories, as shown in **Table 7.4**.

7.3 Phobic anxiety disorders

In these disorders, anxiety is caused by anticipation of, or exposure to, specific situations or objects. The patient usually knows that their fears are irrational, but is nevertheless significantly affected and tends to avoid the trigger. Phobic anxiety disorders include agoraphobia, social phobia and specific (isolated) phobias.

Agoraphobia

Agoraphobia (Greek: *fear of the market place*) is a fear of situations that are difficult to escape from (rather than a fear of open places).

Psychiatric	Organic
Affective disorders	Cushing's disease
Personality disorders	Hypoglycaemia
Psychotic disorders	Hyperthyroidism
Eating disorders	Phaeochromocytoma
	Substance intoxication and withdrawal

Table 7.3 Psychiatric and organic contributors to anxiety

Type of anxiety	Symptoms
Psychological	Fear Feeling of impending doom Poor concentration Irritability Exaggerated startle response Restlessness Depersonalisation and derealisation
Somatic	
General	Tremor Headache Aches and pains Sweating, flushes, chills Dizziness Paraesthesia Insomnia
Cardiovascular	Palpitations Tachycardia Chest pain
Respiratory	Tight chest Shortness of breath Hyperventilation
Gastrointestinal	Nausea Butterflies Loose stools Dry mouth Globus hystericus (the feeling of a lump in the throat) Abdominal pains, dyspepsia
Genitourinary	Urinary frequency Amenorrhoea Erectile dysfunction

Table 7.4 Symptoms of anxiety

Clinical features

The patient may be fearful of leaving their home alone, entering crowded places or travelling alone. Avoidance is characteristic, and some people may become housebound.

It is usually seen with panic disorder and social phobia; depressive symptoms and obsessive features may also be present.

Approach to the patient

Possible screening questions for agoraphobia and social phobia (see below) include:

- 'Do you find yourself feeling anxious in particular situations?'
- '… perhaps when leaving the house alone/travelling/in crowded places/when speaking in public/in social situations?'
- 'How does the fear or anxiety affect your life?'
- 'Do you go out of your way to avoid this situation?'

Management

Treatment may involve CBT, with specific behavioural techniques such as graded exposure. Antidepressant medication, such as a selective serotonin reuptake inhibitor (SSRI), may also be useful.

Prognosis

Relapse is common.

Social phobia

People with social phobia experience anxiety in social situations (e.g. public speaking, parties), in which they fear humiliation and embarrassment.

Clinical features

Those with social phobia may avoid triggering situations, possibly leading to employment and social difficulties. Self-medication through alcohol (or benzodiazepine) abuse is common.

Particular symptoms include:
- blushing
- nausea
- hand tremor
- urgency of micturition or defaecation
- panic attacks

Management

Treatment may involve antidepressants, and CBT techniques such as graded exposure. β-Blockers can be useful for the physical symptoms.

Prognosis

There is a high risk of relapse on discontinuation of treatment

Specific (isolated) phobias

This is the most common anxiety disorder. Anxiety symptoms are caused by the fear of a specific situation or object.

Clinical features

Exposure to the feared stimulus, such as those in **Table 7.5**, may trigger a panic attack.

Approach to the patient

Possible screening questions for specific phobias include:
- 'Do you have any particular fears or phobias?'
- 'How does the fear affect your life?'
- 'Do you go out of your way to avoid this fear?'

Cause	Phobia
Enclosed spaces	Claustrophobia
Heights	Acrophobia
Darkness	Achluophobia
Animals	Zoophobia
Blood	Haemophobia
Doctors	Iatrophobia
Thunder	Brontophobia
Snakes	Ophidiophobia
Spiders	Arachnophobia

Table 7.5 Examples of specific phobias

Management
The mainstay of management is CBT, such as systematic de-sensitisation, which involves graded (imagined) exposure and relaxation training.

Prognosis
Phobias do not usually improve without treatment, and can persist for many years.

Other anxiety disorders
These include panic disorder, generalised anxiety disorder and mixed anxiety and depressive disorder.

7.4 Panic disorder

Panic disorder, also known as **episodic paroxysmal anxiety**, is characterised by recurrent, abrupt and unpredictable episodes of severe anxiety (panic attacks).

Clinical features
During a panic attack, the anxiety symptoms commonly lead to catastrophic fears of losing control, going mad or of dying, which in turn provokes further anxiety symptoms. This 'vicious cycle' forms the basis of the cognitive–behavioural model of a panic attack (**Figure 7.1**).

Panics attacks have a rapid onset, reach a peak within 15 minutes, and usually subside after 30 minutes.

Approach to the patient
The diagnosis of panic disorder is based on at least one unexpected panic attack comprising at least four somatic symptoms, plus either marked worry of further attacks or avoidance behaviour.

Possible screening questions for panic attacks include:
- 'Have you ever suddenly felt really anxious or scared … perhaps with your heart beating rapidly, your hands shaking, or you were sweating a lot?'
- 'What were you doing at the time?'
- 'How often does it happen?'

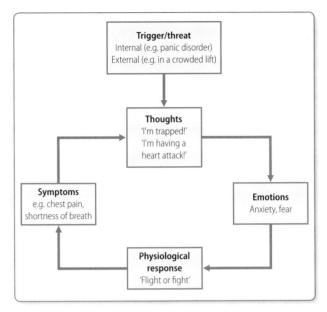

Figure 7.1 Cognitive–behavioural model of a panic attack.

Management

CBT is a particularly effective treatment in panic disorder. Antidepressants (such as SSRIs) and self-help groups may also be used. Benzodiazepines are not recommended in panic disorder, owing to the high risk of dependence.

> **Clinical insight**
>
> Panic attacks occur not only in panic disorder but also in depressive disorders, generalised anxiety disorder, social phobia, medical conditions (e.g. hyperthyroidism) or substance misuse.

7.5 Generalised anxiety disorder

GAD is characterised by persistent anxiety without a clear trigger, with disproportionate worry about ordinary situations across various life areas.

Clinical features

Somatic symptoms, such as muscle tension, headache, dizziness, tremor and palpitations, are common.

Anxiety, depression and medical disorders are often coexistent, and attempts to self-medicate may lead to substance misuse.

Those with GAD may struggle with their work and social functioning.

Approach to the patient

Possible questions to ask regarding GAD include:
- 'Have you found yourself worrying a lot recently?'
- 'What is it that you worry about?'
- 'Do your worries interfere with your life?'

Management

Treatments include CBT, self-help and self-help groups, psychoeducation, applied relaxation and drug treatment with SSRIs, serotonin–norepinephrine reuptake inhibitors (SNRIs) and, more recently, pregabalin.

Prognosis

GAD tends to be chronic and disabling, especially if there is a comorbid anxiety disorder or depression.

7.6 Mixed anxiety and depressive disorder

This diagnosis is used to describe the presence of both anxiety and depressive symptoms that are insufficient to fulfil the criteria for either depressive disorder or an anxiety disorder.

7.7 Obsessive–compulsive disorder

A person with OCD may have predominantly obsessional thoughts or compulsive actions, or a mixed presentation.

Epidemiology

OCD usually develops in early adulthood, and may be precipitated by a traumatic event. Exacerbations can be linked to stress.

OCD affects both genders equally.

Causes/pathogenesis

There is probably a genetic contribution, but no specific genes have been identified.

OCD is associated with anankastic personality disorder, depression, Tourette's syndrome and Sydenham's chorea (St Vitus' dance).

The last two indicate abnormalities of the basal ganglia being central to the pathogenesis. This is supported by imaging and functional studies, which suggest that pathology of the caudate nucleus results in an abnormal signalling loop between the orbitofrontal cortex and the thalamus.

Alterations in serotonergic and dopaminergic neurotransmission also appear to be involved.

Clinical features

Obsessional thoughts are uncontrollable images, ideas or impulses that occur repeatedly despite attempted resistance.

- The content may be obscene, violent or otherwise taboo, and therefore usually distressing, particularly if the person fears they may act on their impulses
- The person recognises them as their own thoughts (cf. thought insertion)
- Sometimes they may consist of endless doubts that impede decision-making

Compulsive acts are pointless, stereotyped behaviours, which the person is compelled to repeat in order to allay a subjective fear.

- The fear is often that harm will come to themselves or a loved one should they resist
- The person usually knows that their 'rituals' are useless, and gain no pleasure from them (cf. autistic spectrum disorders)

- Acts commonly involve cleaning (e.g. hand washing), tidying or keeping objects orderly/symmetrical, or checking (e.g. gas hobs/front door); they may persist for hours at a time

Approach to the patient

Possible screening questions for OCD include the following.

For **obsessional thoughts**:

- 'Do certain things keep coming into your mind, even though you try to keep them out?'
- 'What effect is this having on your life?/How are you coping with this?'
- 'Do you sometimes find it difficult to make decisions, even small ones?'
- '… perhaps because there seem to be too many options?'

For **compulsive actions**:

- 'Do you find yourself spending a lot of time doing the same thing over and over again, even though you have already done it properly?'
- 'Why do you feel that you need to do this?'
- 'What happens if you try to stop doing this?'

Management

Management strategies for OCD include self-help groups, CBT and antidepressants (e.g. SSRIs).

Exposure and response prevention is a particular form of CBT used to help people with OCD to master their obsessions or compulsions. The person is repeatedly exposed to their feared scenario, and assisted to cope with – rather than avoid – their anxiety until the anxiety response ceases.

Prognosis

The course of OCD is often chronic. Secondary depression, anxiety or substance misuse may develop.

An acute trigger, employment and episodic course point towards a better prognosis; a worse outcome is more likely with an early onset, longer duration, the presence of depression or need for symmetry.

7.8 Stress and adjustment disorders

These include acute stress reaction, post-traumatic stress disorder and adjustment disorders.

Acute stress reaction

A transient disorder occurring almost immediately after extreme physical and psychological stress (e.g. near-death experiences) in vulnerable individuals.

Clinical features

An acute stress reaction consists of a mixture of varying symptoms, including:

- some clouding of consciousness, inattention and disorientation ('shock')
- withdrawal and avoidance
- somatic features of panic

In extreme responses, it may lead to dissociative fugue or stupor (see Dissociative/conversion disorders).

The symptoms may subside in hours, and certainly within a few days, after which there may be total amnesia for the episode.

Management

Often, explanation, reassurance and support is all that is required for management.

Post-traumatic stress disorder

With historical terms including 'shell-shock' and 'combat neurosis', PTSD was first described after the Vietnam War. It is a protracted or delayed response to a extremely threatening or catastrophic experience.

Clinical features

These include:

- flashbacks (repeated intrusive memories)
- nightmares
- autonomic overarousal with hypervigilance and a heightened startle response

- detachment
- numbness/emotional blunting
- avoidance of reminders
- anhedonia

Comorbidities, such as substance misuse, anxiety and depression, are common.

Management

Management includes:
- medication, e.g. SSRIs
- psychological therapies, e.g. trauma-focused CBT (CBT principles are applied to the past trauma, and used to explore the related memories, emotions and behaviour)

> ### Clinical insight
>
> **Eye movement desensitisation and reprocessing** (EMDR) is a post-traumatic stress disorder treatment used in some centres, the efficacy of which has been demonstrated but the method of action remains unknown.
>
> In EMDR, the patient attends to a neutral visual stimulus (e.g. the therapist's moving fingers) while concentrating on recollected images, sensations, thoughts and negative emotions connected to their trauma. The process is repeated , emphasising particularly challenging memories. Eventually (8–12 regular sessions), the patient becomes sufficiently comfortable with the painful images to be able to recall them at the same time as an associated positive thought.

Debriefing, the routine discussion of traumatic events soon after they occur, is **not** recommended.

Prognosis

The majority of those with PTSD recover, although enduring symptoms and personality change can occur in a minority.

Adjustment disorders

Adjustment disorders are periods of distress in response to a significant life change or traumatic life event, such as the loss of a relationship, migration or retirement. Abnormal bereavement (grief) reaction falls within this group.

Clinical features

Symptoms include a low mood, anxiety, worry and a subjective inability to cope or plan ahead. The symptoms impede normal day-to-day functioning, but do not fulfil the diagnostic criteria of other conditions, e.g. depression.

Management/prognosis

Intervention is not usually required, and the prognosis is good.

7.9 Medically unexplained symptoms

Medically unexplained symptoms (MUS) are real symptoms for which **current** medical science affords no clear cause. The aetiology is often assumed to be psychological in nature.

MUS are very common, accounting for possibly:

- 30% of presentations to GPs
- 15% of presentations to cardiology clinics (e.g. non-cardiac chest pain)
- 50% of presentations to gastrointestinal clinics (e.g. irritable bowel syndrome)

When these symptoms are particularly severe, perhaps significantly impeding a patient's normal functioning, a referral may be made to a psychiatrist.

MUS include dissociative conversion disorders and somato-form disorders.

Dissociative/conversion disorders

Historically referred to as 'hysteria', the ICD-10 definition of these disorders describes a 'partial or complete loss of the normal integration between memories of the past, awareness of identity and immediate sensations, and control of bodily movements'.

Medical examination and investigation do not reveal the presence of any known physical or neurological disorder.

Freud's theory that such presentations are the result of psychological pain being 'converted' into physical symptoms is reflected in the alternative term **conversion disorder**.

Clinical features

Commonly, the history will reveal a recent traumatic event, interpersonal difficulties, or subjectively hopeless problems.

The loss of function seen in dissociative disorder may be a symbolic expression of needs or internal conflicts. For example, it may transpire that a patient who suddenly lost the ability to speak was previously frustrated by her inability to 'speak out' about dysfunctional family relationships.

The symptoms in dissociative disorders often appear suddenly, and correspond to how the patient believes a physical illness to present.

Those with dissociative/conversion disorders characteristically portray *'la belle indifference'*, displaying little regard for objectively severe symptoms (e.g. limb paralysis).

Types: The main forms of dissociative disorder in the ICD-10 are:

- **dissociative amnesia**: discrete loss of memory, often for a traumatic event
- **dissociative fugue**: a person with dissociative amnesia embarks on an uncharacteristic and sometimes prolonged journey, during which their behaviour may appear normal
- **dissociative stupor**: significant voluntary motor retardation and response to external stimuli
- **trance and possession disorders**: transient loss of the awareness of the self and surroundings/replacement of the self with another entity, which is unsought (e.g. not a normal cultural or religious experience)
- **dissociative motor disorders**: may mimic a wide variety of motor disorders, such as ataxia or aphonia, although usually involve paralysis of a limb
- **dissociative convulsions**: 'pseudoseizures' may be similar to those in epilepsy (**which may be coexistent**), but loss of consciousness, secondary injuries, urinary incontinence and tongue biting are unlikely, and serum prolactin is not raised afterwards
- **dissociative anaesthesia and sensory loss**: may accompany motor symptoms. Usually, there is skin sensory loss, perhaps with paraesthesia; loss of special senses is rare

Somatoform disorders

These disorders are characterised by recurrent presentations to doctors with physical symptoms and requests for medical investigations, despite repeated investigations revealing no physical cause to explain the symptoms.

The symptoms are experienced as real, and patients may understandably become distressed by their perceived lack of treatment. Comorbid depressive and anxiety disorders commonly occur, especially with hypochondriacal disorder.

Clinical features

Somatoform disorders in ICD-10 include somatisation disorder, hypochondriacal disorder, somatoform autonomic dysfunction and persistent somatoform pain disorder.

> ## Guiding principle
>
> In **DSM-IV**, conversion disorder is included within 'somatoform disorders', and includes only the dissociative motor disorders, convulsions and anaesthesia and sensory loss of the ICD-10 classification.
>
> In **ICD-10**, the symptoms of dissociative disorders include a loss of sensation and problems with physical functions usually under voluntary control. Symptoms involving pain and autonomic functions fall under somatisation disorder.

Somatisation disorder: Also known as **Briquet's syndrome**, this consists of at least two years of numerous variable and recurring unexplained physical symptoms. These result in characteristically complex hospital records, and in a reduction in functioning.

Hypochondriacal disorder: A lasting fear of having a serious illness, despite medical evidence to the contrary. Patients may have somatic symptoms or complain about their appearance.

Somatoform autonomic dysfunction: This involves worry about a physical disorder of a body system under autonomic control, based on autonomic or non-specific symptoms.

Persistent somatoform pain disorder: This is unexplained chronic severe pain that can be assumed to be related to psychological/social problems.

Differential diagnoses

The differential diagnoses include factitious disorder and malingering (**Table 7.6**).

Disorder	Description	Notes
Dissociative/conversion disorder	Dissociation between usually integrated mental processes/'conversion' of psychological symptoms into physical symptoms	May be a lack of concern for apparently severe symptoms
Somatoform disorder	Physical symptoms unattributable to another physical/psychiatric disorder	Includes conversion disorders in DSM-IV
Factitious disorder	Deliberate falsification of symptoms in order to adopt the sick role	Also known as Münchhausen syndrome
Malingering	Deliberate falsification of symptoms in order to achieve a goal other than adopting the sick role, e.g. gaining benefit payments or avoiding prison	Not a psychiatric condition

Table 7.6 Comparison between dissociative, somatoform and factitious disorders, and malingering

Guiding principle

As can be seen, there is considerable overlap between dissociative/conversion and somatoform disorders. This reflects, in part, the lack of an evidence-based pathogenesis.

Management

Following appropriate medical investigations, the management of somatoform disorders involves a clear, supportive explanation to the patient. They require a certain degree of acceptance, but the risk of iatrogenic harm must be emphasised.

Graded exercise, pain rehabilitation, CBT and psychodynamic psychotherapy may be useful in individual cases.

Substance misuse

8.1 Clinical scenario

Confusion and visual hallucinations

Presentation

36-year-old Jack has been brought into the psychiatric unit under Section 136 of the Mental Health Act (1983) of England and Wales. After being alerted to a man wandering next to a busy road, the police found him 'confused', 'paranoid' and possibly responding to visual hallucinations.

There is no record of any previous psychiatric history, though he is known to the police after being apprehended twice for attempted shoplifting of alcohol from his local supermarket.

Diagnostic approach

There is a wide differential diagnosis, but the report of confusion and visual hallucinations means that organic illness must first be excluded.

History

Jack is unkempt, with facial erythema and a distended abdomen. He is sweating with dry lips and a productive cough. Holding his hands over his eyes, protecting them from the ceiling lights, he is only relaxed once they are turned down.

Rapport is difficult to establish. He is agitated, irritable and appears suspicious of the staff. He is preoccupied with 'spiders', which he sees crawling over the floor and over his body. He repeatedly picks up these 'spiders' from the floor, staring intently at his coarsely tremulous hands.

The few limited answers he provides make it clear that he is disorientated in place and time, and cannot recall recent events. He fearfully declines a glass of water, accusing staff of trying to poison him. As a nurse takes it out of the room, the door slams shut and he puts his hands over his ears.

Diagnostic approach

Jack is delirious, and it is likely that he is dependent on alcohol. A coherent history has so far been elusive, but several clinical observations point towards **delirium tremens,** namely his disorientation, psychomotor agitation, amnesia of recent events, persecutory thoughts, visual hallucinations and high sympathetic tone (coarse tremor and sweating).

He is at risk of complications, including seizures and death, and requires prompt treatment in a general hospital.

Next steps include vital observations and a physical examination; a blood sugar reading and other blood tests; and treatment with chlordiazepoxide, vitamins and necessary fluids and antibiotics.

8.2 Alcohol

Alcohol has been drunk by people of various cultures for thousands of years. In 2009, 85% of adults in the UK reported drinking alcohol. In appropriate quantities, it provides pleasure and possibly a reduced risk of death from heart disease. In excess, however, it is associated with significant health and social problems. In the UK it was recently estimated by the Department of Health that:

> You have to begin to lose your memory, if only in bits and pieces, to realise that memory is what makes our lives. Life without memory is no life at all …
>
> Luis Buñuel
>
> (Quoted in Oliver Sachs, *The Man Who Mistook his Wife for a Hat*, regarding a patient with Korsakoff's syndrome)

- 7% of all hospital admissions are alcohol related
- up to 70% of weekend emergency department presentations are alcohol related
- harmful use of alcohol costs the UK National Health Service (NHS) approximately £2.7 billion per year

Guiding principle

The alcohol content of a drink is measured in units: 1 unit = 8 g (or 10 ml) of alcohol (the amount in half a pint of average strength beer, a small glass of wine or a single measure of spirits).

The UK government's recommended limits for alcohol consumption are:

- Men: three to four units a day, up to 21 units a week
- Women: two to three units a day, up to 14 units a week

The problems caused by alcohol, or other substances, exist over a spectrum, but there are several defined stages on this spectrum (**Table 8.1**).

Epidemiology

According to the WHO global statues report on alcohol and health, 2011:

- the harmful use of alcohol results in 2.5 million deaths worldwide every year
- alcohol consumption is the third largest global risk factor for disease and disability

In England, approximately 10 million people are thought to drink above the recommended guideline levels. According to the NHS Information Centre for Health and Social Care, in 2007, alcohol dependence affected 6% of men and 2% of women (or 1.1 million people).

As problem drinking is common, significant and treatable, routine screening of people for alcohol misuse is useful. This is true within all clinical specialties.

Screening questionnaires

A simple and brief test is the **CAGE** questionnaire:

Stage	Details
Intoxication	An acute, transient state of characteristic physical and mental effects caused by consuming the substance
At-risk or hazardous use	The stage between normal and harmful use
Harmful drinking	Substance use is causing damage to the person's physical or mental health, or to their functioning
Dependence	A set of physical and psychological features as defined in ICD-10 and DSM-IV (see Diagnostic criteria)
Withdrawal	A transient, characteristic state which may follow abrupt abstinence from a substance to which the person has developed a tolerance or dependence

Table 8.1 Stages of substance abuse

C Have you ever felt that you should Cut down on your drinking?

A Have you been Annoyed by others criticising your drinking?

G Have you ever felt Guilty about your drinking?

E Have you ever had an (Eye opener) drink first thing in the morning?

Two or more positive answers indicate alcohol abuse.

A superior test for hazardous and harmful drinking is the longer **AUDIT** (Alcohol Use Disorders Identification Test), developed by the World Health Organization and in the UK recommended as the 'gold standard' by the National Institute for Health and Clinical Excellence. It has 10 questions, each with a varying number of possible answers and associated points. The person's drinking can be classified, according to the points scored, as low risk, hazardous, harmful or possible alcohol dependence.

Causes
Genetics

Although the exact genetic mechanisms are unclear, there is strong evidence that alcohol dependence is partly hereditary:

- concordance rates for alcohol dependency in monozygotic twins are significantly higher than in dizygotic twins
- first-degree relatives of alcohol-dependent people are at least twice as likely as controls to develop alcohol dependence themselves
- children of alcohol-dependent parents continue to have an increased personal risk even after adoption by healthy parents

Psychological

There is an association between alcohol/drug misuse and certain personality types, in particular emotionally unstable personality disorder, antisocial personality disorder and childhood conduct disorders.

Psychological theories regarding alcohol and drug abuse include:

- copying (modelling) role models, peers or society as a whole

- positive reinforcement: pleasant effects leading to repeated use
- negative reinforcement: unpleasant effects lead to avoidance
- conditioning: formation of an association between circumstances (pub/needles) and a conditioned response (drinking/using drugs)

Social

Higher rates of drinking tend to be seen in men, the young and those with lower educational levels and in lower socioeconomic groups. Certain types of occupation also increase the risk, including publican, travelling salesman, entertainer and doctor.

The risk of alcohol dependence may be increased by significant life events, such as bereavement, separation and loss of employment.

Comorbidities

The term **dual diagnosis** is used to describe the presence of both a psychiatric disorder and separate substance misuse in a person. Depressive, anxiety and stress disorders, as well as chronic pain and terminal illness, increase the risk of alcohol misuse and dependence. Alcohol problems can, in turn, lead to other psychiatric illnesses and numerous medical conditions (see Clinical features).

Symptoms of anxiety and depression in a person with alcohol dependence commonly resolve on cessation of drinking. This should be kept in mind when considering antidepressant use.

Guiding principle

The metabolism of alcohol involves the oxidation of ethyl alcohol by **alcohol dehydrogenase** to acetaldehyde, which itself is oxidised to carbon dioxide and water by **acetaldehyde dehydrogenase**.

East Asian populations are less likely to develop alcohol dependence because they have an isoenzyme of aldehyde dehydrogenase that leads to an accumulation of acetaldehyde on drinking alcohol and unpleasant symptoms such as flushing, palpitations, nausea and headache.

Alcohol as a drug

Alcohol exerts several effects on the central nervous system:

- anxiolytic properties from an increase in γ-aminobutyric acid (GABA) activity
- amnesia from a decrease in glutaminergic transmission
- euphoria from dopamine release

Reward pathways Certain brain connections are thought to have a role in mediating pleasurable effects and the motivation to obtain further pleasurable stimuli (**Figure 8.1**).

Clinical features

The patient may present in any stage of the following states.

Intoxication

The effects of acute alcohol intoxication are well known to the majority of people. They can include:
- euphoria and relaxation
- disinhibition
- impaired judgement

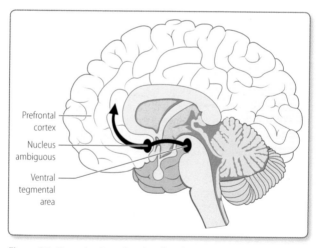

Prefrontal cortex

Nucleus ambiguous

Ventral tegmental area

Figure 8.1 'Reward pathways' are thought to be involved in substance misuse. Connections between the midbrain ventral tegmental area, the nucleus accumbens in the limbic system (the so-called 'pleasure centre') and prefrontal cortex are thought to act as reward pathways

- impulsiveness
- lability of mood
- aggression
- cerebellar effects, e.g. slurred speech, ataxia, nystagmus

Higher blood alcohol concentrations can lead to stupor and coma.

Withdrawal

Withdrawal symptoms range from mild to life-threatening. Uncomplicated effects occur several hours after drinking, often on waking and may last for up to five days without treatment or further drinking:

- sweating
- nausea and vomiting
- tachycardia
- insomnia
- coarse tremor
- anxiety and agitation
- transient hallucinations/illusions
- craving

Grand mal seizures complicate up to 10% of withdrawals, usually one to two days after the last drink; 5% of people develop the medical emergency delirium tremens.

Complications

Delirium tremens This has an untreated mortality of around 10%. It usually occurs one to three days after drinking is reduced or stopped. The risk of developing it is increased by a past history of delirium tremens or withdrawal seizures, concurrent infection or pre-existing liver pathology.

Delirium tremens is distinguished from uncomplicated withdrawal by a clouding of consciousness (delirium). Other signs include:

- disorientation
- suggestibility
- psychomotor agitation
- amnesia for recent events
- insomnia
- fear

- persecutory delusions
- auditory, visual and tactile illusions/hallucinations
- adrenergic overactivity: tremor, sweating, hyperthermia, tachycardia and hypertension may lead to cardiovascular collapse
- seizures

Wernicke–Korsakoff syndrome Wernicke's encephalopathy and Korsakoff's psychosis/Korsakoff amnestic syndrome result from neurodegeneration secondary to **thiamine deficiency**. As their aetiology and occurrence are linked, they are described together as Wernicke–Korsakoff syndrome. Most commonly, thiamine deficiency is due to a chronic high alcohol intake, but can have other causes, such as starvation and malabsorption.

Wernicke's encephalopathy is an acute medical emergency. Wernicke described it as a triad of:

- acute confusion
- ataxia
- ophthalmoplegia (commonly abducens)

Not all of these may be present. Other possible signs include nystagmus and peripheral neuropathy.

Korsakoff's psychosis develops in around 70% of patients with Wernicke's encephalopathy. It is also known (more precisely) as **amnesic syndrome**, as patients have an irreversible inability to form new memories, often leading them to **confabulate** (the falsification of memory in clear consciousness). These 'memories' may be firmly held.

Approach to the patient

Always ask permission before enquiring into people's substance use. Be sensitive with your questions, gathering all the key details without being demanding. Avoid being judgemental and chastising of their actions.

Some people will be reluctant to divulge their drink or drug habits. They may feel guilty, unwell, depressed or suspicious of your intentions (e.g. to tell the police about their heroin use, or the theft required to pay for it). They may be pessimistic about recovery, perhaps after previous unsuccessful attempts.

Alcohol history

Establish the patient's intake on a typical day:

- type(s) of alcohol
- amount: be as precise as possible, use alcohol units
- time
- place, who with?

If there is no such 'typical day', ask about an average week, or about the last time they drank. Assess the effect of their drinking and the possibility of change with further questions, covering:

- The features of alcohol dependence (see Diagnostic criteria)
- Lifetime history of alcohol use
- Any previous treatment/contact with alcohol services
- Past medical history: any significant comorbidities?
- Effects of alcohol on health:
  - mental health, e.g. depression, anxiety, suicidal thought or deliberate self-harm
  - physical health: e.g. gastritis/peptic ulcer, pancreatitis, liver disease
  - diet and nutrition
- Other effects of alcohol on their life:
  - family and relationships
  - employment
  - financial
  - any issues with the police
  - accidents
  - driving
- Any other substances used
- Attitude to drinking and the harm it may be causing
- Motivation to change: what do they wish to achieve, and why?

After the history, explain how their consumption compares with the recommended limits. Discuss the management options available, offering your recommendations, but remembering that any plan needs to be shared and realistic. Avoid either trivialising the problems or being overly authoritative.

Investigations

Blood tests are insufficiently sensitive or specific for screening of alcohol problems, although they can have a role in monitoring consumption (**Table 8.2**).

Diagnostic criteria

Alcohol dependence

The ICD-10 and DSM-IV require **at least three** features from lists similar to that below, in order to make a diagnosis of alcohol dependence:

- primacy of drinking over other activities
- compulsion to drink; a strong desire or craving
- uncontrolled drinking; unable to control starting, stopping or amounts
- tolerance to alcohol; larger doses are required to obtain the same effect
- withdrawal symptoms on stopping or reducing intake; may require a relief drink
- persistence with drinking despite harm
- stereotyped pattern of consumption
- reinstatement after abstinence

Test	Notes
γ-glutamyl transferase (GGT)	Raised in 60–80% of people with alcohol dependence and up to 50% of heavy drinkers Also raised by other forms of liver disease, and pancreatic pathology
Mean corpuscular volume (MCV)	Raised in around 50% of heavy drinkers Also raised by low vitamin B_{12}/folic acid, liver disease, thyroid abnormalities
Carbohydrate deficiency transferrin (CDT)	The most specific test, but is not routinely available

Table 8.2 Blood tests to monitor for alcohol use

Management
Hazardous or harmful drinking

Structured brief advice This should be offered initially; if this is insufficient, extended brief intervention can be used.

Brief intervention should use the FRAMES model, and result in a joint management plan with practical tips for achieving set goals, e.g.

- drinking targets
- seeking help from others
- being aware of avoidable cues for drinking (e.g. stress or drinking partners)
- exploring coping strategies

The **FRAMES** model for brief intervention (NICE 2010):

- **F**eedback (on the patient's risk of alcohol-related problems)
- **R**esponsibility (change is the patient's responsibility)
- **A**dvice (clear advice provided when requested)
- **M**enu (discuss the options for change)
- **E**mpathy (warm, reflective and understanding approach)
- **S**elf-efficacy (optimism about the behaviour change)

Extended brief intervention involves a series of supportive but challenging motivational interviews to assist the person in addressing and reducing their alcohol use to low-risk levels, or abstinence.

Alcohol dependence

Alcohol dependence requires detoxification and support to maintain abstention.

Detoxification This can be carried out in the community, but may require a hospital admission, especially with:

- a history of seizures or delirium tremens
- comorbid medical or psychiatric conditions
- poor social support

Detoxification is achieved with a reducing dose of the benzodiazepine **chlordiazepoxide**, typically over five to seven days.

Intravenous thiamine is given concurrently, with oral B vitamins prescribed in the longer term.

Maintenance Abstention after detoxification has a better prognosis than controlled drinking. Long-term follow-up is crucial for achieving this.

Pharmacological interventions for aiding maintenance include:

- **acamprosate**: 'anti-craving' action
- **disulfiram**: sensitising – concurrent alcohol consumption leads to unpleasant flushing, tachycardia, headache and nausea
- **naltrexone**: opiate antagonist – specialist use only

Psychological interventions include:

- structured groups (run by community alcohol teams, or other organisations e.g. Alcoholics Anonymous); prolonged contact with others treated for alcohol dependence is important for maintaining abstinence
- cognitive–behavioural therapy
- marital or family therapy

Delirium tremens

Management involves emergency detoxification with benzodiazepines. In addition, intravenous thiamine (vitamin B_1) should be given, fluid and electrolyte abnormalities corrected and coexistent infections sought and treated.

Wernicke–Korsakoff syndrome

This can be prevented with thiamine supplementation for those at risk. Once Wernicke's encephalopathy has developed, it is treated with intravenous thiamine, but unfortunately only 20% recover and mortality is over 10%.

Clinical insight

Alcohol and pregnancy: the best advice is to avoid drinking completely when pregnant, as any safe level of consumption remains unknown. Alcohol abuse increases the risk of stillbirths and other obstetric complications, such as **fetal alcohol syndrome:**

- mid-facial abnormalities
- growth retardation
- learning disabilities
- impulsiveness

Complications/prognosis

Alcohol dependence is a chronic, relapsing condition. Up to 70% of people relapse within six months of treatment for alcohol misuse. Comorbid mental illness, poor motivation, unemployment and a lack of social support are risk factors for a worse prognosis.

Other psychiatric sequelae of harmful alcohol use

These include:

- depressive disorder
- anxiety disorders
- suicide and deliberate self harm
- increased risk of violence in schizophrenia
- alcoholic hallucinosis: rare; follows chronic heavy alcohol use and often resolves with abstinence. Usually auditory hallucinations when sober – which progress from sounds to derogatory voices over time
- Othello syndrome/pathological jealousy: delusions of the infidelity of a partner. Potentially significant risk of harm to others. Treated with abstinence and antipsychotic medication

Medical complications

For medical complications, see **Table 8.3**.

Social complications

These include:

- family and relationship difficulties
- criminal activity
- unemployment
- homelessness

8.3 Drugs

Throughout history, human-kind has sought mind-altering substances. Societal and cultural views on these have varied greatly, and they continue to do so. Many governments continue to 'wage war' on the £200

> ... thou hast the keys of Paradise, oh, just, subtle, and mighty opium!
>
> Thomas De Quincey
>
> *Confessions of an English Opium-Eater*

Type	Complication
Neurological	Wernicke–Korsakoff syndrome
	Head injury and subdural haematoma (from trauma)
	Peripheral neuropathy
	Seizures
	Cerebellar degeneration
Neoplastic	Cancers of the bowel, breast, liver, mouth and oesophagus (the risk of the last three is increased further by smoking)
Gastrointestinal	Alcoholic hepatitis
	Liver cirrhosis: around 20% of alcohol-dependent people
	Oesophageal varices
	Pancreatitis: acute and chronic
	Gastritis and peptic ulcers
Cardiovascular	Hypertension
	Cardiomyopathy
	Arrhythmias
	Stroke
Other	Increased risk of infections
	Vitamin deficiencies
	Erectile dysfunction
	Fetal alcohol syndrome
	Accidents

Table 8.3 Medical complications of harmful alcohol use

billion illicit trade, while at the same time use is being increasingly medicalised. Meanwhile, in some societies, drugs maintain traditional roles in ceremonies and rituals.

Table 8.4 shows the classification of drugs controlled under the UK's Misuse of Drugs Act 1971. The major types of illegally used drugs are described below.

Opioids

Opiates, such as the opium alkaloids morphine and codeine, and the semisynthetic heroin, are derived from the opium

Class	Drugs in class
A	Ecstasy, LSD, heroin, cocaine, crack, magic mushrooms, amphetamines (if prepared for injection)
B	Amphetamines, cannabis (reclassified from C in 2009), methylphenidate (Ritalin), pholcodine
C	Tranquilisers, some painkillers, γ-hydroxybutyrate, ketamine

Table 8.4 UK classification of controlled drugs. Source: www.homeoffice.gov.uk.

poppy. The opioid group also includes fully synthetic compounds, such as pethidine and methadone.

Heroin (**Figure 8.2**) was originally produced in 1896 as an analgesic, and named as the hero of medicines. It continues to be commonly prescribed, by its scientific name diamorphine, for pain relief and acute pulmonary oedema. As a drug of abuse, heroin may be snorted, smoked (chased), or injected intravenously, subcutaneously (skin popping) or intramuscularly.

Street names Smack, gear, brown and skag.

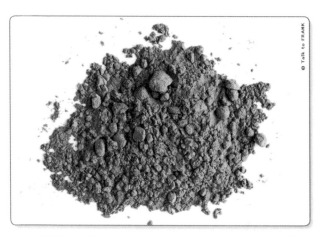

Figure 8.2 Heroin. The opium poppy was known to the Sumerians over 4000 years ago as the 'joy plant'. Courtesy of FRANK (a UK national drugs helpline)

Cannabis

Cannabis comes in various forms (**Figure 8.3**), such as dried leaves (marijuana/grass/weed), resin (hash) and cannabis oil. Skunk is a particularly strong form of cannabis. Cannabis can be smoked in spliffs or joints (usually with tobacco) or a bong (water pipe), eaten (perhaps in a cake) or drunk as an infusion.

Street names Marijuana, pot, dope, weed, grass, ganja, green and hash.

Cocaine

The stimulant effects of the coca leaf were known to the indigenous people of South America before cocaine was isolated in the nineteenth century. Cocaine (**Figure 8.4**) is usually snorted, although it can be smoked or injected in the form of crack cocaine (also known as freebase cocaine owing to the removal of hydrochloride to increase effect).

Street names Charlie 'C', coke and snow.

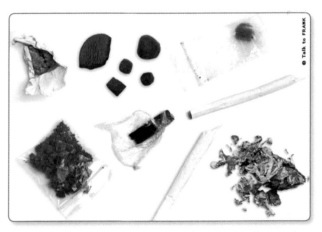

Figure 8.3 Cannabis is derived from the *Cannabis sativa* plant. Courtesy of FRANK (a UK national drugs helpline)

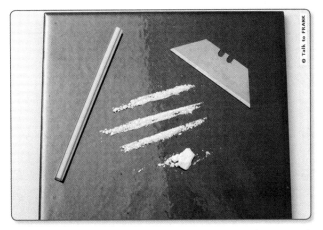

Figure 8.4 Cocaine: until 1914, this was an ingredient in Coca Cola. Courtesy of FRANK (a UK national drugs helpline)

Amphetamines

This class includes methamphetamine (meth, crystal meth), dexamphetamine (speed) and ecstasy (see below). Methylphenidate (Ritalin) is a treatment for attention deficit and hyperactivity disorder. Amphetamines (**Figure 8.5**) are usually swallowed as tablets. They can also be smoked or injected intravenously, as with the 'ice' form of methamphetamine.

Street names speed, whizz, ice, uppers, dexies, billy, meth, crystal meth and ice.

Ecstasy

Also known as MDMA, ecstasy (**Figure 8.6**) was synthesised early in the twentieth century.

Street names 'E', disco biscuits, XTC, vitamins, eccies and pills.

Hallucinogens

This group includes LSD (lysergic acid diethylamide), PCP (phenycyclidine) and magic mushrooms.

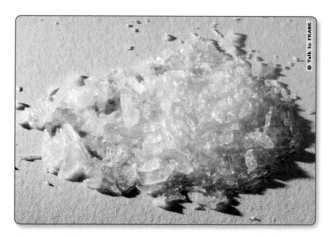

Figure 8.5 Methamphetamine, used by soldiers in the Second World War.
Courtesy of FRANK (a UK national drugs helpline)

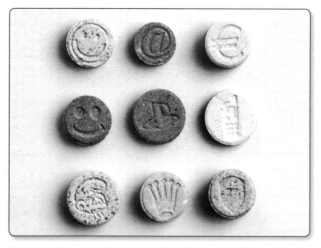

Figure 8.6 Ecstasy was first synthesised in the early twentieth century.
Courtesy of FRANK (a UK national drugs helpline)

Street names Acid, tabs and trips.

Benzodiazepines
These prescribed medications (see Chapter 2) are also drugs of abuse.

Volatile substances
The effects of these substances, such as glues, gases and aerosols, are achieved through inhalation of their vapours.

Epidemiology
Drug use in England and Wales in 2009/10
The following information is taken from the NHS Statistics on Drug Misuse (2010).
Overall use:
- 8.6% of adults (16–59 years) used one or more illicit drug: 6.6% used cannabis, 3.1% used class A drugs
- 20% of young adults (16–24 years) used one or more illicit drug: 16.1% used cannabis, 7.3% used class A drugs

Admissions to hospital for drug-related mental health and behavioural disorder (England only):
- 5809 people as primary diagnosis (70% male)
- 44,585 people as primary or secondary diagnosis (67% male)

Contact with drug treatment services:
- 206,889 people aged over 18 years (73% male)

Discharges after treatment for drug dependency:
- 62,685 people in total: 38% were no longer dependent; 15% were referred for further interventions; 47% dropped out or discharged for other reasons

Problematic drug use is mostly associated with the young, but substance misuse in older people should also be considered, especially with bereavement, social isolation or chronic illness/pain.

Causes
There is much overlap with the risks factors for alcohol misuse.

Cannabis has been focused on as a 'gateway drug': as the most common drug for initial experimentation, it may lead to use of other substances. The likelihood of this first step is increased when drugs are more readily available and more accepted within the peer group.

Clinical features
Heroin

Mechanism All opioids act on opioid receptors, the target of endogenous peptides known as endorphins (endogenous morphine). Heroin is a particular agonist of μ (mu) opiate receptors in the brain and spinal cord.

Effects These include:
- immediate euphoria
- sedation
- analgesia
- pinpoint pupils
- constipation, anorexia, nausea
- bradycardia
- pruritus

Overdose This leads to respiratory depression and coma; aspiration of vomit is a common cause of death in overdose. Management of an overdose involves supportive measures and the administration of intravenous naloxone, an opioid antagonist.

Most heroin users become dependent, usually progressing from smoking to regular intravenous use. Tolerance builds easily, and some users may merely aim to avoid withdrawal symptoms. After abstinence, tolerance rapidly diminishes, leaving the user at a high risk of overdose should they begin again with their last dose.

Withdrawal The process of withdrawal from heroin is unpleasant but, unlike withdrawal from alcohol, it is not usually dangerous. It begins some 6–12 hours after last use, peaking between 36 and 72 hours, and lasting 7–10 days. Commonly referred to as 'cold turkey' owing to the symptoms of chills and piloerection, it is also marked by:

- intense craving
- abdominal discomfort
- muscle pain
- insomnia
- restlessness
- yawning
- pupillary dilatation
- various 'leaks' or 'runs'; diarrhoea, vomiting, lacrimation and rhinorrhoea

Management A careful history, and urine drug screen, should be used to confirm opioid use before prescribing a substitute medication.

Psychological and social support should be offered alongside medication use.

If abstinence is a realistic option, then detoxification using a substitute agent such as methadone or buprenorphine can be carried out:

- the drug is stopped and the substitute prescribed at a gradually reducing dose (at least initially under supervision)
- abstinence can be aided with naltrexone, a long-acting opiate antagonist
- care should be taken to ensure the patient is no longer dependent; otherwise, naltrexone would induce withdrawal

If abstinence is unrealistic, then harm reduction strategies can be used instead.

Longer term maintenance prescribing of substitute medication can allow some people to stabilise their drug use and lifestyles.

Other interventions include advice on safer drug use, such as avoiding intravenous and lone drug use, the provision of clean needles, and prevention of, testing for and treatment of blood-borne and sexually transmitted diseases.

Clinical insight

Naloxone has a usefully rapid action. The sudden reversal of opioid effects may not, however, be appreciated by a patient abruptly removed from their euphoric state!

Also, its short half-life means that the patient needs to be closely monitored for the return of opioid effects after administration.

Cannabis

Mechanism The key component is Δ-9-tetrahydrocannabinol, which acts on brain cannabinoid receptors.

Effects These can vary according to the mood of the user. There may be:
- alterations in aesthetic experiences and the perception of space and time
- sometimes euphoria; others can become paranoid and anxious
- impaired reaction time and motor skills
- red eyes, dry mouth, tachycardia
- increased appetite (the 'munchies')

Long-term use of cannabis can lead to depression, anxiety, low motivation, an increased risk of psychosis and the health problems associated with smoking.

Overdose This may lead to confusion and psychosis.

Withdrawal This is a controversial concept. It is more common in long-term users. It consists of usually mild anxiety, restlessness and irritability. Dependence is uncommon.

Management This involves advice on reducing or stopping use.

Cocaine

Mechanism Cocaine acts by blocking the reuptake of serotonin, dopamine and noradrenaline.

Effects These include:

Clinical insight

Crack cocaine is named after the sound of the rocks burning.

- euphoria
- increased confidence and energy, and less need for sleep or food
- dilated pupils, tachycardia, hyperthermia and hypertension
- paranoid ideation and aggression
- auditory and visual hallucinations; classically formication.

Chronic use can lead to nasal septum necrosis, anxiety and psychosis.

Overdose This can be fatal. Its features are:

- confusion
- psychosis
- cardiac arrhythmias
- respiratory arrest
- stroke
- seizures

Guiding principle

The short-lived cocaine high and subsequent unpleasant 'crash' can lead to repeated, sometimes compulsive, use. Crack generates a more intense but even shorter high, and has significant rates of dependence.

Management of overdose involves symptomatic and supportive measures, and possibly benzodiazepines and antipsychotics for psychosis.

Withdrawal Symptoms include craving, dysphoria (feeling ill at ease), anxiety, irritability, agitation, fatigue, hypersomnolence, suicidal ideation and vivid dreams.

Management There is no cocaine substitute, so management consists primarily of harm reduction strategies. Advice can be given on reducing or stopping use, and any comorbidities should be treated.

Amphetamines

Mechanism Amphetamines, like cocaine, block the reuptake of monoamines such as noradrenaline and dopamine, although they have a longer half-life.

Intoxication This results in:

- increased energy
- insomnia
- anorexia
- tachycardia, hypertension and hyperthermia

Clinical insight

Chronic heavy use of amphetamines can lead to stereotyped repetitive behaviours, and a schizophrenia-like psychosis.

- sometimes dysphoria, anxiety, irritability and confusion

Overdose This can cause:

- cardiac arrhythmias and cardiovascular collapse
- severe hypertension and stroke
- seizures
- coma

Management of an overdose involves the appropriate supportive measures and symptom management.

Withdrawal Symptoms include:

- craving
- dysphoria
- fatigue
- depression and suicidal ideation
- anxiety
- nightmares

Management This takes the form of harm reduction strategies. Advice can be given on reducing or stopping use, and any comorbidities should be treated.

Ecstasy

Mechanism Ecstasy increases serotonin release while inhibiting its reuptake.

Effects Intoxication leads to the typical effects of a stimulant, along with increased sociability and feelings of closeness with others. Users can also experience:

- teeth grinding (bruxism)
- sweating
- nausea
- hyperthermia, dehydration and excessive consumption of water (with subsequent electrolyte disturbance) can lead to death

Overdose Ecstasy can cause similar problems to those of amphetamines.

Withdrawal This consists of a dysphoric and fatigued 'comedown'.

Management This involves harm reduction strategies, such as avoiding hyperthermia and dehydration.

Hallucinogens

Mechanism These cause alteration of serotonergic and dopaminergic activity.

Effects Hallucinogens lead to 'trips' of distorted sensory experiences and sometimes synaesthesia (see **Chapter 1**). Some people have a 'bad trip', with anxiety and distress. Dangerous behaviour, such as attempting to use delusional powers of flight, can occur.

Overdose This is unusual, but can cause autonomic overactivity, nausea and vomiting, hyperthermia and coma.

Withdrawal This does not seem to oc cur, although unpleasant flashbacks can occur years later.

Management This takes the form of harm reduction.

Benzodiazepines

Benzodiazepines (also see **Chapter 2**) can be taken orally or injected. Their in-

> ### Clinical insight
> Benzodiazepine overdose, which may lead to respiratory depression, is managed using flumazenil, a benzodiazepine antagonist.

toxication, overdose and withdrawal effects are similar to those of alcohol. Dependence is common, and unfortunately it is often iatrogenic, following incautious prescriptions.

Management This involves detoxification or maintenance prescribing using benzodiazepines with longer half-lives, or harm reduction strategies such as education and appropriate prescribing.

Volatile substances

Mechanism These cause increased GABA-ergic activity.

Effects Intoxication is rapid, and similar to that of alcohol. There may be hallucinations.

Overdose Adverse and overdose effects include cardiac arrhythmias, central nervous system and other organ damage, asphyxia, coma and death from aspiration.

Withdrawal There are not usually any effects, but headaches and fatigue may follow use.

Management: The aims are harm reduction and promotion of abstinence.

Complications/prognosis
Drug misuse tends to run a chronic, relapsing and remitting course.

Complications
Complications of intravenous drug use include:
- local infections
- venous thrombosis
- systemic infections such as bacterial endocarditis, HIV, and hepatitis B and C
- emboli

Harm to pregnancy
The effects of using illicit drugs in pregnancy are not fully known, but none have been proved to be safe, and therefore avoidance of all is advised. Cocaine is reported to increase the risk of a low-birthweight, premature birth, and childhood behavioural problems. Heroin is reported to increase the risk of a low birthweight, and withdrawal symptoms in the newborn.

Comorbid psychiatric conditions
Depression, anxiety disorders and personality disorders are common in drug use, which can act as a precipitating and perpetuating factor.

Social problems
These include:
- relationship difficulties
- unemployment
- criminal activity

Organic psychiatry: delirium and dementia

chapter
9

Traditionally, psychiatric conditions have been divided into functional and organic disorders. Organic disorders were thought to result from identifiable pathological lesions, medical disorders and drugs. Functional disorders were thought to result from a change in 'functioning' of the brain. Schizophrenia, bipolar affective disorder and depression were thus all considered functional. This division was clearly an oversimplification, with many functional disorders now having identifiable neuropathological features. History and current research indicate that almost all disorders have biological, psychological and social contributions.

The main organic disorders encountered are delirium and dementia, and these shall be the focus of this chapter. **Table 9.1** shows some other organic conditions and their psychiatric presentations.

9.1 Clinical scenario

A forgetful 71-year-old

Presentation

The following referral is received: Thank you for seeing Ernest, a 71-year-old man, who lives with his daughter. His wife passed away last year. Both Ernest and his daughter are concerned that he has become increasingly forgetful. He forgets having started tasks such as boiling a kettle and on leaving the house sometimes forgets where he is going. His appetite and sleep are poor. There is a past history of depression around 10 years ago for which he was treated with an SSRI. Otherwise he is in good physical health.

Diagnostic approach

More information is needed from a careful history and mental state examination. Collateral history is particularly relevant

Neurological conditions	
Stroke	Effects depend on site of lesion Personality change, emotional lability, behavioural problems and dementia are common Post-stroke depression affects ~35% Entire spectrum of psychiatric disorders can be seen
Cerebral neoplasm	Effects depend on the site of lesion, e.g. frontal tumours causing behavioural changes, occipital tumours and visual hallucinations ~50% have psych symptoms on presentation
Epilepsy	Very high frequency of psychiatric symptoms, e.g. déjà vu, hallucinations, depersonalisation and amnesia Increased prevalence of all common psychiatric disorders and self-harm
Multiple sclerosis	Personality change, mood disturbance and cognitive deficits
Parkinson's disease	Non-motor symptoms greatest cause of morbidity Treatment of motor symptoms may cause psychosis Depression in ~50%
Endocrine conditions	
Hypothyroidism	Common: cognitive impairment, mental slowing and depression seen commonly Rare: 'myxoedema madness' (dementia, delirium and psychosis) seen rarely
Hyperthyroidism	Anxiety and irritability are common features together with weight loss May also cause mania or delirium
Cushing's disease	Depression common in addition to weight gain, insomnia and loss of libido. Psychosis may occur
Addison's disease	Depression (50%), mild cognitive impairment (50%), apathy, tiredness (80%) and anorexia
Phaeochromo-cytoma	Prominent anxiety
Hypercalcaemia	Delirium, psychosis, cognitive impairment and depression common presenting features
Other conditions	
HIV	Wide spectrum of psychiatric symptoms Depression affects 30–50% at some point with 30-fold increased suicide risk 30% AIDS patients develop HIV-associated dementia Psychosis with atypical features

Table 9.1 Key organic conditions and their psychiatric manifestations

as the patient may not be able to give a complete account of events. In elderly patients, depression can present with cognitive decline. This is pseudodementia and should improve on treatment of the depression. It will be important to assess the duration of symptoms.

Within the mental state examination, cognitive function is particularly relevant and typically a screening tool such as the mini-mental state examination (MMSE) would also be used. Physical health assessment is needed to exclude delirium. The differential diagnosis remains wide but higher possibilities include **depression**, **dementia** (type unknown) and **delirium**.

Initial history

Between the referral and time that he is assessed, there appears to have been a marked deterioration in the patient. He is slow and has a slight tremor. His daughter mentions that he has had three falls and, on one occasion, banged his head. She says that are periods when he seems completely fine, but today is not one of those; in fact, she was concerned that he experienced some hallucinations the previous night. She first noticed the memory problems about a year ago.

Diagnostic approach

This information emphasises the value of a collateral history. The long-standing nature of memory problems indicates dementia. The fluctuating course, presence of hallucinations, tremor and bradykinesia are suggestive of **Lewy body dementia**. Nonetheless, recurrent delirium and depression remain a possibility and he may have sustained a subdural haematoma during the falls. Other intracranial pathology, such as normal pressure hydrocephalus or neoplasm, may have been responsible for the falls.

Further history

Ernest appears older than his age, is poorly shaven and using a stick. His attention to conversation appears normal and there is no clouding of consciousness. He is, however, irritated by questioning. His speech is slightly stuttering. Apart from reduced appetite and poor sleep, there is nothing to indicate depression. He confirms seeing animals in his room the night before but has good insight. An MMSE is carried out to assess his cognition and he scores 20.

Physical examination reveals some bruising from falls, cogwheel rigidity, bradykinesia and a resting tremor but little else. His gait is normal and there is no history of urinary incontinence.

Diagnostic approach

Depression and delirium now appear less likely. The working diagnosis should be Lewy body dementia; however, routine blood tests should still be performed to exclude reversible causes of dementia. These turn out to be normal. Neuroimaging should be performed and may include a specialised single photon emission computed tomography (SPECT) scan to specifically assess for the reduced dopaminergic transmission seen in Lewy body dementia. Full psychosocial assessment is required before creating a holistic management plan, which may include medication in the form of an acetylcholinesterase inhibitor.

9.2 Delirium

Also known as 'acute confusional state', ICD-10 defines delirium as 'an acute, transient and global disorder of brain function resulting in disturbance of consciousness and attention, thinking, memory, psychomotor behaviour, emotion and the sleep wake cycle.' It should be viewed as a sign that something untoward is occurring physically. Whenever someone, especially an elderly person, presents with an acute change in mental state, it must be considered. The duration is variable and the degree of severity ranges from mild to very severe.

Epidemiology

Delirium is a common disorder affecting approximately 14–24% of all hospital inpatients and over 30% of geriatric inpatients. It has been estimated to account for 49% of all hospital days.

Causes

Predisposing factors for delirium include increasing age, dementia, a past history of delirium, poor functional status, sensory impairment, poor oral intake, polypharmacy and multiple medical conditions. **Table 9.2** outlines some of the more common causes.

Clinical features

There is rapid onset clouding of consciousness. findings on mental state examination include:

- behavioural changes which can be both hyperactive with agitation, aggression and wandering (difficult to miss) or hypoactive with drowsiness and withdrawal (easy to miss)
- speech is often incoherent and rambling
- mood is labile with anxiety, perplexity and irritability most common

Type of cause	Cause
Neurological	Ischaemic stroke, subarachnoid haemorrhage, head injury, space-occupying lesions, epilepsy (including post-ictal state), any other condition causing cerebral hypoperfusion
Metabolic	Any disorder causing electrolyte imbalance (renal failure, hepatic failure, cardiac failure, dehydration, malnutrition)
Endocrine	Hypoglycaemia, diabetic ketoacidosis, thyroid dysfunction, Cushing's syndrome
Infective	Urinary tract infection, pneumonia, cellulitis, encephalitis, endocarditis, meningitis, septicaemia, HIV, malaria, tuberculosis
Drugs	Alcohol, analgesics (especially opiates), sedatives, anticholinergcs, diuretics, corticosteroids, anticonvulsants, lithium, tricyclic antidepressants, monoamine oxidase inhibitors, L-dopa
Other	Hypoxia, anaemia, arrhythmias, sleep deprivation, urinary retention, faecal impaction, postoperative, vitamin deficiencies including thiamine, pain

Table 9.2 Common causes of delerium

- sleep disturbance is often seen and symptoms are frequently worse at night
- there are perceptual disturbances such as misidentification, delusions and hallucinations
- there is a reduced ability to maintain attention and memory is impaired with poor registration and retention
- delirium can mimic most psychiatric disorders to the untrained eye

Symptoms of the underlying cause may or may not be present.

Table 9.3 highlights the features differentiating delirium and dementia.

Investigations

Physical examination and investigations are a priority. Investigations include:

- blood tests: full blood count (FBC), erythrocyte sedimentation rate (ESR), urea and electrolytes (U&Es), liver function tests (LFTs), thyroid function tests (TFTs), Ca^{2+} level, iron studies, lipid profile, vitamin B_{12}, folate, glucose and blood cultures

Feature	Delirium	Dementia
Onset	Acute/subacute	Chronic, insidious
Course	Fluctuating	Stable but progressing
Duration	Days to weeks	Months to years
Consciousness	Altered	Clear
Attention	Markedly impaired	Normal/slightly impaired
Delusions (if present)	Fleeting	Systematised
Hallucinations	Common	Less common (except Lewy body dementia)
Psychomotor activity	Usually abnormal ($\uparrow$ or $\downarrow$)	Usually normal
Sleep–wake cycle	Disturbed	Usually normal

Table 9.3 Differentiating delirium and dementia

- urine microbiology
- ECG
- chest radiograph
- other: depending on the clinical findings and investigation results: abdominal radiograph, CT/MRI, HIV testing, electro-encephalogram (EEG)

Management
General
Delirium is usually managed in a general hospital or nursing home setting with any treatment being given under common law. In exceptional circumstances, the terms of mental health legislation may need to be employed to give treatment. After initial assessment and basic investigation, the following behavioural measures should be implemented:

- regular observation
- nurse in a side room
- address sensory problems, e.g. glasses, light levels, hearing aids
- avoid excessive changes, e.g. transferring between wards, changing nurses, changing doctors, changes to daily routine
- attempt to orientate the patient, e.g. through regular conversation, use of clocks, calendars, photos of family
- remove hazardous objects
- encourage safe mobilisation and exploration of the environment
- avoid physical restraints

Medical
The following medical measures should also be implemented:

- identify and treat the underlying cause
- stop unnecessary medications
- maintain fluid and electrolyte balance
- medication: avoid sedation unless absolutely required (i.e. severely agitated or posing a risk). Low-dose haloperidol is usually the agent of choice and can be given orally or intramuscularly. Atypical antipsychotics can also be used. Benzodiazepines may be useful if there is a component of

alcohol withdrawal or if sleep is the main problem; note, however, that generally they have been shown to prolong and sometimes worsen delirium

> **Clinical insight**
>
> Do not expect delirium to resolve as soon as a physical cause has been treated; it can take days or even weeks.

- monitor recovery with regular clinical review including serial abbreviated mental test score (AMTS)/MMSE testing

Complications/prognosis

Delirium is associated with increased mortality both in the short term (approximately 10% per episode) and in the longer term, with 1-year mortality of 35–40%. Delirium also leads to longer inpatient admissions and an increased likelihood of nursing home placement.

9.3 Dementia

Dementia is a clinical syndrome characterised by difficulties in memory, disturbances in language, psychological changes and impairment in the ability to perform activities of daily living. It can be caused by a wide variety of disease processes.

Epidemiology

Worldwide, approximately 24.3 million people have dementia. This number is expected to rise to 81.1 million by 2040. In the UK, 650,000 people have a dementia syndrome and the annual cost of their care is £17 billion; this compares with £4 billion spent on the care of patients with heart disease and £2 billion on those with cancer.

Dementia is one of the main causes of disability in later life, contributing 11.2% of all years lived with disability, compared with 9.5% for stroke, 8.9% for musculoskeletal disorders and 2.4% for cancer. Its prevalence increases with age (**Table 9.4**). A comparison of the risk factors and epidemiology of common types of dementia is shown in **Table 9.5**.

Age (years)	Prevalence
80+	1 in 5
70–80	1 in 20
65–70	1 in 50
40–65	1 in 1000

Table 9.4 UK prevalence of dementia by age group

Causes

Dementia can be classified as primary or secondary, but in reality the aetiology can be mixed (**Table 9.6** and **Figure 9.1**).

Some of the causes are reversible, e.g. vitamin deficiencies, endocrine abnormalities and subdural haematomas.

Clinical features

The symptoms vary depending on the cause (**Table 9.7**).

Common symptoms can be remembered as the 'five As':

- **amnesia**: Loss of memory starting with short-term memory, impaired learning and disorientation
- **apraxia**: Loss of the ability to carry out skilled tasks, e.g. washing and dressing
- **agnosia**: Visuospatial difficulties, inability to recognise faces (prosopagnosia), illusions
- **aphasia**: Expressive and receptive dysphasia/aphasia
- **associated** features:
  - behavioural disturbance: wandering, sleep, sexual disinhibition, aggression
  - anxiety and depression: common but needs to be looked for and as in children on basis of behaviour at times
  - Delusions: affect 20-40%. They are typically paranoid in quality, e.g. regarding theft, persecution and infidelity
  - hallucinations: affect 50% in Alzheimer's disease; almost all in Lewy body dementia

Type	Epidemiology	Risk factors
Alzheimer's disease (AD)	Commonest cause (~45%) 500,000 people in UK Prevalence doubles every 5 years from the age of 65 Women slightly more affected	1. Age 2. Genetics **Early onset** often familial, associated with rare autosomal dominant mutations which alter β-amyloid metabolism. include presenilin 1 and β-APP (chromosome 21) **Late-onset** is associated with inheritance of the ε4 allele of apolipoprotein E. ε2 allele is protective 3. Family history 4. Head injury 5. Low IQ 6. Low socioeconomic status 7. Obesity and diabetes
Vascular dementia	25% of dementias Higher prevalence in countries such as Japan (~50%) May present with AD Men>women	1. Age 2. Vascular risk factors hypertension, diabetes, obesity, hypercholesterolaemia, smoking, atrial fibrillation 3. Family history
Lewy body dementia (LBD)	~15% of dementia Onset slightly earlier than AD	1. Age 2. Family history 3. Parkinson's disease
Fronto-temporal dementia (Pick's disease)	<5% of all dementias Women affected more than men Earlier onset, typically 45–60	1. Family history in 50% of cases 2. Genetics: up to 50% of cases are caused by mutations of MAPT or PGRN genes
Huntington's disease	Population prevalence: 4–7 per 100,000 Men and women equally affected Onset in 30s/40s but may be earlier	Autosomal dominant neurodegenerative disorder Results from CAG trinucleotide repeats encoding glutamine in the Huntingtin gene on chromosome 4 Genetic anticipation: higher # CAG repeats = lower age of onset

Table 9.5 Comparison of the epidemiology and risk factors of common dementias. APP, amyloid precursor protein.

Primary (degenerative)	Alzheimer's disease Dementia with Lewy bodies Frontotemporal dementias Huntington's chorea
Secondary	Vascular: vascular dementia, subarachnoid haemorrhage
	Inflammatory, including demyelinating: multiple sclerosis, systemic lupus erythematosus, arteritis Infections: encephalitis, meningitis, HIV/AIDS dementia, syphilis, prion diseases
	Neoplastic: primary or secondary tumours, paraneoplastic syndrome
	Metabolic: chronic vitamin deficiencies (vitamin B_{12} and thiamine), cardiac, hepatic, renal failure, chronic anaemia
	Endocrine: hypothyroidism, parathyroid disorders, hypopituitarism, Addison's disease, Cushing's syndrome
	Trauma: severe head injury, 'punch-drunk' syndrome/dementia pugilistica, subdural haematoma
	Drugs and toxins: chronic alcohol use, carbon monoxide poisoning, exposure to heavy metals such as lead, mercury and aluminium
	Miscellaneous: normal pressure hydrocephalus, epilepsy (usually severe and chronic)

Table 9.6 Primary and secondary causes of dementia

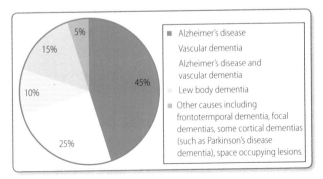

Figure 9.1 Causes of dementia and their prevalence (UK data)

Type	Neuropathology	Clinical features
Alzheimer's disease (AD)	Extracellular β-amyloid plaques Intracellular neurofibrillary tangles Loss of cholinergic neurones Initial cortical atrophy in temporal and parietal lobes CT: widened sulci, shrunken gyri, enlarged ventricles and atrophied temporal lobes	Insidious onset and gradual progression of memory loss and personality change 5 'A's: Amnesia Apraxia Agnosia Aphasia Associated features
Vascular dementia	Cystic necrosis of infarcted areas Reactive gliosis CT: ischaemic changes, especially periventricular ischaemia, multiple infarcts	Sudden onset with stepwise decline Personality change Focal neurological signs Evidence of vascular disease elsewhere, e.g. peripheral
Lewy body dementia (LBD)	Lewy bodies in cortical and subcortical neurones Neuronal loss leading to cholinergic deficit and other neurotransmitter abnormalities CT: relative sparing of medial temporal lobes. SPECT scanning can be used to confirm diagnosis (reduced dopaminergic transmission)	Fluctuation in cognitive impairment and alertness Visual hallucinations and other psychotic symptoms Parkinsonism (tremor, rigidity, bradykinesia) Sensitivity to neuroleptics Frequent falls and faints
Fronto-temporal dementia (Pick's disease)	'Ballooned' neurones called Pick cells Tau-positive inclusions called Pick bodies Gliosis and atrophy affecting frontal and temporal lobes CT: characteristic 'knife-blade' atrophy of the frontal and temporal lobes	Early personality change, especially disinhibition Dementia with prominent frontal lobe symptoms Speech disturbances Apathy/restlessness Memory can be preserved in early stages Primitive reflexes re-emerge

Contd...

Huntington's disease	Abnormal huntingtin protein causes the degeneration of neurons	Psychiatric symptoms present first, including depression and psychosis
	Caudate nucleus, putamen and cerebral cortex most notably affected	Choreiform movements
		Dementia
	CT: atrophy of basal ganglia and dilation of ventricles	

Table 9.7 Comparison of the pathology and clinical features of common dementias. CT, computed tomography; SPECT, single photon emission computed tomography.

Approach to the patient

When assessing the patient:

- have a high index of suspicion in elderly patient groups
- a good patient and collateral history are the most important part of diagnosis

It may be useful to ask friends and family about:

- forgetfulness or anxiety about forgetfulness
- difficulties outside the patient's normal routine
- change in personality
- change in activities or hobbies and reason why
- word-finding difficulties
- duration of onset: gradual/stepwise or sudden

Cognitive assessment

The MMSE is used most commonly, although other screening instruments exist such as the AMTS, General Practitioner Assessment of Cognition and the Six-Item Cognitive Impairment Test.

Mini-mental state examination: This takes approximately 20 minutes to complete and can be used to estimate the severity of impairments and monitor the course of cognitive changes. It assesses orientation, attention, immediate recall, short-term memory, naming of common objects, following of simple verbal commands, following of simple written commands and copying a figure. The test is scored out of 30. A score of less than 25 indicates dementia; 10–20 would indicate moderate dementia; and less than 10 indicates severe dementia. Remember that other factors can affect performance and the sensitivity is relatively low, meaning that it is no replacement for thorough history.

Physical examination and investigations

Physical examination and investigations are vital to assist diagnosis and exclude potentially reversible causes. Initial investigations are blood tests, serology, neuroimaging, EEG, chest radiograph, ECG, urine testing and lumbar puncture.

Blood tests These include FBC, ESR, U&Es, LFTs, TFTs, Ca^{2+} level, iron studies, lipid profile, vitamin B_{12}, folate and glucose.

Serology Patients should be tested for syphilis (Venereal Disease Research Laboratory test) and HIV if indicated.

Neuroimaging This may include:
- CT to exclude intracranial lesions; cerebral infarction and haemorrhage; extradural and subdural haematomas; normal pressure hydrocephalus
- MRI, which provides higher resolution and can show focal atrophy for example
- SPECT to assess regional blood flow
- a radioisotope ioflupane (^{123}I) uptake scan with SPECT to detect Lewy body disease

Further neuropsychological testing should also be carried out to assess specific deficits.

Electroencephalogram (EEG) This should be carried out if epilepsy or encephalopathy are suspected.

Much as with cancer or other severe medical condi-

> ## Clinical insight
>
> The benefits of early diagnosis of dementia include:
> - treatment of reversible physical and psychiatric causes
> - treatment of comorbid conditions and risk factor reduction
> - initiation of psychosocial support and pharmacological interventions
> - planning for the future while still competent to do so
> - avoiding 'crises'

tions, careful consideration must be given to breaking news of the diagnosis.

Differential diagnoses

The differential diagnosis is initially between the primary and secondary causes of dementia, as listed in **Table 9.6**.

Other conditions to consider include:
- delirium (**Table 9.3**)
- depression: this can commonly cause poor concentration and memory, especially in the elderly, and hence is referred to as pseudodementia
- late-onset schizophrenia

Management

General principles

The treatment and prognosis of common types of dementia is given in **Table 9.8**. A biopsychosocial approach to the management of dementia is outlined in **Table 9.9**.

Management is increasingly co-ordinated through memory clinics, which usually operate in parallel with older adult community mental health teams and perform the following functions:
- diagnosis and access to specialist investigations such as neurocognitive assessment and neuroimaging
- access to multidisciplinary assessment and interventions, e.g. occupational therapy and social services
- medication prescribing and monitoring
- education, training and support for carers
- knowledge of appropriate local care provision
- access to charities
- monitoring for complications
- co-ordinating admission to hospital if required

Medication

Acetylcholinesterase inhibitors, such as donepezil, galantamine and rivastigmine, are used in Alzheimer's disease and Lewy body dementia. These act by preventing the breakdown of acetylcholine, hence increasing neurotransmitter levels to compensate for the overall loss of cholinergic neurones. The N-methyl-D-aspartic

Type	Treatment	Prognosis
Alzheimer's disease (AD)	General measures Acetylcholinesterase inhibitors NMDA receptor antagonists (memantine)	Progressive deterioration Life expectancy ~8 years from time of diagnosis
Vascular dementia	General measures Vigorous treatment of vascular risk factors	Stepwise deterioration Shorter life expectancy than for AD
Lewy body dementia (LBD)	General measures Cholinesterase inhibitors Avoid antipsychotics	Life expectancy ~6 years from time of diagnosis
Fronto-temporal dementia (Pick's disease)	General measures Highly sensitive to psychotropic medication	Life expectancy ~8 years
Huntington's disease	General measures Antipsychotics may help reduce abnormal movements	Life expectancy 14–15 years from onset High suicide rate (~10%)

Table 9.8 Comparison of the treatment and prognosis of common dementias. NMDA, N-methyl-d-aspartic acid.

acid receptor antagonist memantine is also licensed. These drugs do not reverse dementia but may delay further decline. They should only be prescribed by a specialist and need regular review to assess their risk–benefit profile.

Medication may be used to treat comorbid psychiatric illnesses, but should only be used as a last resort in the management of behavioural disturbance. Antipsychotics are associated with an increased risk of stroke.

Complications/prognosis
In summary:
- most dementias progress until death

Short term management	Medium and long term management
Biological Definitive diagnosis Medication: acetylcholinesterase inhibitors if indicated Address modifiable risk factors, e.g. hypercholesterolaemia with statins Treatment of comorbid medical conditions	Regular review Beware of superimposed delirium Treat comorbid psychiatric illnesses Psychotropic medication as a last resort for behavioural disturbance, e.g. trazodone, benzodiazepines, low-dose antipsychotics Rationalise medication as condition progresses Palliative care approach in advanced dementia
Psychological Counselling Psychoeducation Cognitive–behavioural therapy	Bibliotherapy Behavioural analysis, i.e. identifying and modifying triggers for specific behaviours such as wandering due to boredom Reminiscence therapy Snoezelen (controlled multisensory stimulation) rooms
Social Appropriate package of care Discuss risks of driving and need to inform appropriate agency (Driver and Vehicle Licensing Agency, in the UK) Family education Carer support	Patient groups Day centres Charities Benefits Housing Employment Power of attorney Prepare advance directives Carer respite

Table 9.9 General principles of dementia management using a biopsychosocial model

- the average life expectancy from onset is five to eight years and the degree of morbidity is highly variable
- 60% of people with dementia are able to live in their own home, but increasing support will be required

- so-called 'behavioural and psychological symptoms in dementia' are common. These include problems such as wandering, shouting or aggression. Management requires thorough clinical assessment to exclude treatable causes such as infection or pain. Inpatient admission or elderly mentally infirm (EMI) placements may be required
- physical, financial and sexual abuse are relatively common in this patient group and should be monitored for.

Eating, sleep and sexual disorders

chapter

10

10.1 Clinical scenario

Unusual eating habits developing over time

Presentation

Katie is a 15-year-old girl who makes an appointment to see her GP for a physical check-up as she has decided to run a marathon. Her family GP knows that Katie is from a middle class family and has always achieved excellent grades at school.

During a previous consultation Katie's mother had expressed concern that on starting secondary school, her daughter began to experience bullying and teasing by friends for never having had a boyfriend. Her elder sister had suggested that maybe she should wear more make-up and lose a bit of weight, saying "everyone else in the family is thinner than you." Katie had consequently resolved to become a vegetarian and her mother had noticed that she was spending a great deal more time in the bathroom.

The GP notes that Katie looks much younger than her 15 years, is wearing very baggy clothing and looks quite thin.

Diagnostic approach

There are many features here to suggest an eating disorder. The use of a screening tool, such as the **SCOFF questionnaire**. The SCOFF questionnaire (**Table 10.1**) is used as a five-point screening tool for eating disorders by GPs and other non-specialists. A score of 2+ indicates the need for further history and possible referral. It may be helpful in deciding whether or not to refer for specialist input

At assessment, an understanding of the patient's own body image should be reached, BMI calculated and a physical examination carried out, paying particular attention to possible physical complications of an eating disorder (**Table 10.2**).

1.	Do you ever make yourself **S**ick because you feel uncomfortably full?
2.	Do you ever worry you have lost **C**ontrol over how much you eat?
3.	Have you recently lost more than **O**ne stone in a 3-month period?
4.	Do you believe yourself to be too **F**at when others say you are too thin?
5.	Would you say that **F**ood dominates your life?

Table 10.1 the SCOFF screening questionnaire.

Initial history

During the consultation, Katie refuses to be weighed; however, she does report that her periods have stopped. The GP refers her to a psychiatrist. She does not attend.

A year later she collapses while at school and is taken to hospital, where her weight is found to be just 30 kg; being 154 cm tall, her BMI is 12.6.

> **Clinical insight**
>
> To calculate body mass index (BMI):
> $$BMI = Weight\ (kg)/[Height\ (m)]^2$$

Diagnostic approach

Katie requires inpatient admission, ideally to a specialist unit. She most probably fulfils the criteria for a diagnosis of anorexia nervosa. As an inpatient, the aim will be to stabilise her physical health, to achieve weight gain of around 0.5 kg/week through a careful dietary plan and partake in a programme of psychological treatment. There is a risk of refeeding syndrome (severe electrolyte imbalance); therefore, regular blood tests will be required during the initial period.

Indications for admission in eating disorders include:

- rapid or extreme weight loss (>1 kg lost per week or BMI <13)
- electrolyte imbalance (typically $\downarrow K^+$, $\downarrow Na^+$, $\downarrow PO_4^{3-}$)
- temperature <34.5°C; pulse <45 beats per minute; blood pressure <80/50
- change in mental status due to malnutrition
- cardiac complications/other acute medical disorder
- long-term failure of outpatient treatment

System	Complications and findings
Electrolytes	Varied presentation depending on patient characteristics; typically $\downarrow K^+$, $\downarrow Na^+$, $\downarrow PO_4^{3-}$ Requires close monitoring during refeeding
Cardiovascular	Bradycardia Hypotension/postural hypotension Mitral regurgitation ECG: arrhythmias, prolonged QTc Blood tests: hypercholesterolaemia
Gastrointestinal	Constipation Abdominal pain (secondary peptic ulceration, oesophageal tears, etc.) Delayed gastric emptying and decreased colonic motility

Endocrine and reproductive	Amenorrhoea
	Infertility
	Reduced libido
	Blood tests:
	    Low luteinising hormone, follicle-stimulating hormone and oestradiol
	    Low triiodothyronine, low thyroxine
	    Mildly elevated cortisol
	    Increased growth hormone levels
	    Impaired glucose tolerance
	    Relative hypoglyceamia

Physical appearance	Thin, gaunt or emaciated Dry skin Brittle hair Erosion of tooth enamel (perimylolysis) Lanugo hair (fine downy hair on forearms, face and back) Russell's sign Delayed sexual maturation Anaemia Cyanosis Orange appearance (hypercarotinaemia) Cold peripheries Hypothermia Peripheral oedema
Other	Proximal myopathy (manifest as an inability to squat and rise) Osteopenia and osteoporosis Renal failure Vitamin deficiencies, deranged lung function tests Pancreatitis

Table 10.2 Complications and findings in eating disorders, especially anorexia nervosa

Further history

Initially, Katie feels angry that everyone is trying to make her fat and is frustrated by the incessant blood tests. Eventually she gets on well with the psychologist and family therapy is a success.

8 years since the initial presentation to her GP, she is a 23 year old in her final year of medical school. She is in a good relationship and has a BMI of 21. Recently, her boyfriend has noticed some secret binge eating and is surprised when he finds a box of laxatives in her room. She explains this by saying that she has always had a problem with constipation. He also notices that she seems to be making a lot of visits to the dentist yet is a steadfast – even obsessive – brusher of her teeth.

Diagnostic approach

These new features are suggestive of bulimia nervosa. It is not uncommon for people to move between the different types of eating disorder or for problems to re-emerge at periods of heightened stress. Laxative abuse is also common, as are dental problems, which usually result from repeated induced vomiting.

> Nothing matters, so long as I am thin.
>
> Katie, anorexia sufferer
>
> Modern anorexia is the biopsychosocial disorder mirroring a society with specific tensions and contradictions: the bourgeois family, supportive yet suffocating, and all the paradoxical hypocrisies of modern attitudes towards youth, food, femininity, beauty and sexuality are whipped up by the media and by multi-million pound food and style industries
>
> Roy Porter; The Greatest
> Benefit to Mankind

10.2 Eating disorders

The core features include:

- preoccupation and excessive focus on body shape and weight
- significant impairment in psychosocial functioning and/or physical health
- abnormal pattern of dietary intake (restriction or bingeing)
- weight control behaviours (e.g. excessive exercise, induced vomiting, use of laxatives)

Eating disorders are classically divided into anorexia nervosa, bulimia nervosa and atypical eating disorders (**Figure 10.1**), although there is a great deal of overlap and movement between these categories that is likely to be reflected in future diagnostic classifications.

Eating disorders and related behaviours are common in young people. A recent study found that 7.1% of boys and 13.4% of girls displayed disordered eating behaviours, leading to the World Health Organization making this a priority area.

The lifetime prevalence of eating disorders in adults is approximately 0.6% for anorexia nervosa, 1% for bulimia nervosa and 3% for binge eating disorder.

Anorexia nervosa

Epidemiology

Although the prevalence of anorexia nervosa (AN) among males is being increasingly recognised, AN is predominantly a female disorder with a female–male ratio of 10:1. The peak age

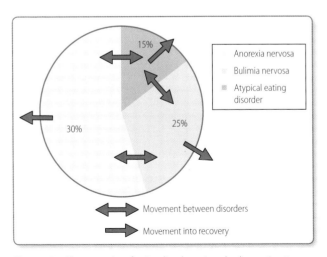

Figure 10.1 The proportion of eating disorder patients by diagnostic category (UK data). Arrows represent movement between disorders and also into recovery

of onset is 16–22 years and lifetime prevalence is 0.6%. There is a possible excess of middle/upper class patients, although all social classes are affected. AN has the highest mortality of any psychiatric disorder and is the most common cause of weight loss in young women.

Eating disorders have been reported worldwide but are rarer in the developing world.

Causes/pathogenesis

The aetiological factors in eating disorders are shown in **Table 10.3**.

Clinical features

AN is a disorder seen mostly in younger women and is characterised by a distorted body image, pathologically low weight and behaviours in the pursuit of thinness.

The four diagnostic criteria are:

1. **Low weight**: weight loss or, in children, lack of weight gain leading to a body weight 15% below normal. BMI is ≤17.5
2. '**Deliberate**' **weight loss**: self-induced weight loss by avoidance of 'fattening foods' together with self-induced vomiting, purging, excess exercising or use of appetite suppressors
3. **Abnormal self-perception** of being too fat with an intrusive dread of fatness, which leads to a self-imposed low weight threshold
4. **Endocrine dysfunction**: widespread endocrine disorder involving the hypothalamic–pituitary–gonadal axis, manifest in women as amenorrhoea and in men as impotence. There is a loss of libido in both sexes and, if the disorder begins before puberty, normal physical development is delayed or arrested

Approach to the patient

A full psychiatric history should be carried out with particular focus on:

Biological	Psychological	Social
Predisposing Female sex Age: adolescence and early adulthood Family history of eating disorder (including obesity), mood disorder, anxiety or addiction Modest evidence of linkage to chromosome 1p Gastrointestinal problems Obesity (bulimia nervosa)	Sexual abuse Family dieting Critical comments about shape or weight from others Altered perception of own body image Low self-esteem Perfectionism	Living in a Western society Adverse parenting (e.g. minimal contact, elevated expectations, marital strife) Occupational or recreational pressure to be slim (e.g. modelling career or gymnast) Affects all social classes
Precipitating –	–	Life stressors such as failed examinations, relationship breakdown or changing school
Perpetuating Starvation itself leading to neuroendocrine changes which perpetuate anorexia	(All of the above)	(All of the above)

Table 10.3 Aetiological factors in eating disorders

- perception of own weight/fear of 'fatness'
- obsessions or rituals surrounding food or mealtimes
- recent weight loss
- food restriction
- purging
- use of appetite suppressants, diuretics and laxatives and excessive exercise

- libido
- menstrual history
- physical health screening questions

Investigations

A full physical examination needs to be carried out, seeking out the medical complications shown in **Table 10.2**.

On first presentation, height, weight and BMI should be recorded and basic blood tests arranged (full blood count, erythrocyte sedimentation rate, urea and electrolytes, thyroid function tests, liver function tests, bone profile, glucose). Consideration should be given to baseline ECG, urinary drug screen, faecal occult blood test and dual energy X-ray absorptiometry (DEXA) bone scans if indicated.

Differential diagnoses

Initially, it is important to consider medical causes of weight loss such as endocrine disorders (e.g. hyperthyroidism, diabetes mellitus, Addison's disease), gastrointestinal disorders (e.g. inflammatory bowel disease, malabsorption syndromes) and other chronic medical conditions (e.g. anaemia, renal failure, cancer).

The more probable differential diagnosis is from psychiatric conditions, primarily from other eating disorders then body dysmorphic disorder, depression, obsessive–compulsive disorder, schizophrenia and personality disorder.

Management

Engagement of the patient and family in treatment is paramount. Initially, this may be at the most basic level of them acknowledging that there is a problem.

A combined approach is then best, involving:

- **psychoeducation**: inform the patient and family about the disorder and its treatment; family members need to learn to be firm but supportive.
- **nutrition**: a plan needs to be negotiated regarding target weight gain (usually 0.5–1 kg/week) and eating regimes; typically, this will involve a dietitian
- **psychotherapy**: family therapy has a strong evidence base in younger patients with a short history whereas interpersonal

therapy may be more appropriate for those in whom the illness is more entrenched; cognitive–behavioural therapy (CBT) is of benefit in addressing perfectionist traits and low self-esteem
- **medication**: should be used **only** to treat comorbid psychiatric or physical disorders

When possible, management should be as an outpatient. Indications for admission include:
- rapid or extreme weight loss (>1 kg lost per week or BMI <13)
- electrolyte imbalance (typically $\downarrow K^+$, $\downarrow Na^+$, $\downarrow PO_4^{3-}$)
- temperature <34.5°C; pulse <45 beats per minute; blood pressure <80/50
- change in mental status due to malnutrition
- cardiac complications/other acute medical disorder
- long-term failure of outpatient treatment

Complications/prognosis

As with all psychiatric disorders, prognosis is variable, with young age and short duration associated with better outcomes whereas psychiatric comorbidity, longer illness duration and purging at low weights are associated with worse outcomes.

If untreated, anorexia has one of the highest mortality rates of any psychiatric disorder (10–15%). Premature mortality of up to 20% is seen in inpatient cohorts.

Overall, 40% will recover (over a 6- to 12-year period); 20% will experience chronic, severe illness or death; the remainder will improve to some extent but retaining abnormal eating habits or develop other eating disorders.

Osteoporosis is a long-term complication and bone recovery takes months to years.

Bulimia nervosa and binge eating disorder

The term bulimia nervosa (BN) is derived from the Greek *bous* (ox) and *limos* (hunger). It was coined in 1979 by Gerald F.M. Russell in his book *Psychological Medicine*, for an illness in which he described overeating as the most consistent feature, often overshadowed by 'intractable self-induced vomiting or purgation'. The clinical diagnosis requires:

- regular episodes of 'binge eating', in which the person may consume enormous amounts of food; typically, those they perceive as being 'forbidden'
- regular episodes of compensatory behaviour; typically, purging follows the binges when feelings of guilt and shame result in efforts to 'undo' the binge, i.e. induced vomiting/use of laxatives. The person does not have to purge, however; instead, they may compensate for binges with periods of severe restriction or excessive exercise
- self-evaluation unduly influenced by body shape or weight
- BMI >17.5

If there is no compensatory behaviour for binges, the diagnosis is one of **binge eating disorder.**

Epidemiology
As with anorexia, BN has a female preponderance, with a female–male ratio of 3:1. Lifetime prevalence among women is 1.5%, and onset is typically during adolescence. Owing to patients often being of normal weight and the typically secretive nature of binges and purges, presentation is often much later than in AN. The aetiology is similar to that seen with AN, although a family or personal history of obesity is more likely. Many will have a previous history of AN or an atypical eating disorder.

Approach to the patient
The prevalence of depressive symptoms is higher than in AN and should be looked out for. Rare neurological syndromes causing overeating such as Kleine–Levin (hypersomnia) and Klüver–Bucy (compulsive orality and hypersexuality) syndromes ought to be considered

Management
It is almost always possible to manage these patients in the community; engagement and education are pivotal early on.
- **medication**: unlike in AN there is a good evidence base for the use of high-dose selective serotonin reuptake inhibitors (fluoxetine 60 mg/day), which ameliorate binging and purging through enhanced impulse control

- **psychotherapy**: CBT should be given as a first-line treatment; interpersonal psychotherapy (IPT) also works, although it takes longer. Both have a robust evidence base
- Treat medical **complications** and psychiatric comorbidities

Prognosis

The prognosis is better than for AN but chronicity is still a problem. CBT and IPT will yield 30–40% remission rates; however, one-third of those with BN followed up long term have an eating disorder 12 years later, and 4% are morbidly obese.

10.3 Sleep disorders

The normal range of sleep varies between 7 and 9 hours for adults, although some can function on as little as 4 hours. Sleep requirements reduce with age by around 30 minutes per decade from middle age.

> Death, so called, is a thing which makes men weep, And yet a third of life is passed in sleep.
>
> Lord Byron

Problems with sleep are extremely common and are one of the major reasons that patients consult their GPs. Sleeping is important. When a person's sleep requirements are not met, daytime somnolence, fatigue, low mood, reduced motivation, worse performance and general decline in quality of life occur.

Classification

Sleep disorders can be divided into

- **primary**: arising directly from a disturbance of the sleep–wake cycle
- **secondary**: arising as a consequence of another psychiatric or medical condition

Terminology

Insomnia is the term used to describe unsatisfactory quantity or quality of sleep.

Hypersomnia refers to excessive daytime sleepiness or prolonged transition between sleep and wakefulness. This is much less common than insomnia and may be caused by other sleep disorders such as narcolepsy or sleep apnoea.

Parasomnias involve abnormal and unnatural movements, behaviours, emotions, perceptions and dreams that occur during sleep (e.g. nightmares, night terrors, somnambulism).

Epidemiology

It is estimated that 5 million people in the UK have a chronic disorder of sleep, but 95% of these remain unidentified or untreated.

Causes

The causes of sleep disorder are shown in **Table 10.4**.

Insomnia

Epidemiology

Insomnia has been estimated to affect one-third of the population during a 1-year period. It is more common in women, the elderly and medical or psychiatric inpatients. Depression and anxiety are thought to underpin over 50% of cases, although insomnia is itself a risk factor for developing depression.

Approach to the patient

History: A thorough history of the problem and general psychiatric and medical history should be obtained. The pattern

Circadian rhythm	Shift work, travel
Neurological	Restless legs syndrome, narcolepsy, brain tumour
Psychiatric	Mood disorders, anxiety, schizophrenia, chronic fatigue syndrome
Behavioural	Poor sleep hygiene
Cardiorespiratory	Obstructive sleep apnoea, chronic obstructive pulmonary disorder, asthma, heart failure
Other medical	Reflux, pain related
Substance or medication related	Alcohol, nicotine, caffeine, prescribed medication

Table 10.4 Aetiological framework for sleep disorders

of sleep disturbance may help to identify the underlying cause. For example, anxiety disorders are associated with difficulty initiating sleep, whereas depressive disorders are characterised by early morning wakening. In hypomania and mania, there is a reduced need to sleep.

Sleep monitoring: Occasionally, sleep diaries, questionnaires, polysomnography (an observed overnight sleep study) or actigraphs (motion sensors) may be required.

Management

The principles of management include:

- treating any underlying cause
- considering the timing of medication with stimulant drugs being given in the morning and sedating drugs at night
- addressing sleep hygiene (see below)
- hypnotics: these are effective but should only be used for short-term treatment (4/52). The duration of action needs to be considered.

> ### Clinical insight
>
> **Hypnotics in sleep disturbance:** Common side-effects include gastrointestinal disturbance, headache, tolerance and dependence. Hypnotics should be avoided in patients with respiratory disease, hepatic/renal impairment and those prone to addiction. Benzodiazepines are the most commonly prescribed, such as temazepam (short acting) and nitrazepam (long acting). Non-benzodiazepine hypnotics, such as zopiclone and zolpidem, are increasingly used whereas melatonin is preferred in children

Sleep hygiene: Advice should be given to:

- limit the use of caffeine to the morning (caffeine has a half-life of five hours), and to avoid alcohol and cigarettes at night
- have a balanced evening meal, not too early or too late
- take regular daily exercise, but avoid late evening exercise
- ensure a comfortable, cool, quiet and dark sleeping environment
- consider the impact of a co-sleeper on your own sleep
- try to maintain a regular routine, avoiding napping during the day or attempting to 'catch up' in the morning
- instigate a relaxing bedtime routine allowing time to wind down before bed. This may include reading, listening to music

or watching television; however, note that looking at computer screens reduces melatonin production and therefore sleep onset
- avoid going to bed until drowsy and ready to sleep
- get out of bed if not asleep within 15–20 minutes and return only when drowsy. This way, the bed is associated with being asleep rather than having difficulty in getting to sleep

10.4 Sexual dysfunction

Sexual disorders can be divided into:
- **sexual dysfunction**, which can be defined as a persistent or episodic impairment of the normal pattern of sexual interest and/or response that interferes with a sexual relationship and causes distress
- disorders of sexual preference and gender identity

Sexual dysfunction is a common consequence of psychiatric disorders and their treatment, e.g. loss of libido in depression or retrograde ejaculation due to antipsychotic drugs. It may also be contributing to the aetiology of a psychiatric disorder

Classification

Sexual dysfunction can be categorised as shown in **Table 10.5.**

Aspect of sexuality affected	Men	Women
Sexual interest	Reduced or excessive sexual desire	Reduced or excessive sexual desire
Arousal	Erectile dysfunction	Sexual arousal disorder (e.g. vaginal dryness)
Orgasm	Premature ejaculation Retarded ejaculation	Anorgasmia
Other	Dyspareunia	Vaginismus Dyspareunia

Table 10.5 Types of sexual dysfunction

Epidemiology

Women: Approximately 10% of women consider themselves to have a problem, although only a fraction of them seek help. The most common problem is low sexual desire. Presentation is generally to the GP or in gynaecology clinics.

Men: The most common dysfunction is premature ejaculation; however, erectile dysfunction (ED) is the main reason for seeking medical advice. ED affects <1% of men under 30, but >25% of those over 70.

Causes

Physical causes of sexual dysfunction are considered in **Table 10.6**; however, sexual dysfunction generally arises from a mixture, and interaction, of psychological and physical causes. It is helpful to consider the problem by listing the predisposing, precipitating and maintaining factors, as in **Table 10.7**.

Approach to the patient

When obtaining a history:
- Talk to both partners
- Determine the nature of problem. Has it always been there or is it new? Is it intermittent or constant? How often do they have sex? What is the nature of that sex?
- **Men**: ask about interest, subjective level of arousal, morning erections, getting/sustaining erections, duration before ejaculation, worry about sexual performance

Cause	Examples
Cardiovascular	Arteriosclerosis, hypertension
Neurological	Spinal cord transection, prolapsed intervertebral disc
Genitourinary	Infection, Peyronie's disease, priapism
Endocrine	Diabetes, hypogonadism
Surgery or accidents	Post prostatectomy, mastectomy, oophrectomy, episiotomy, rectal resection, aorto-iliac surgery, fractured pelvis
Drugs	Antihypertensives, diuretics, antidepressants, neuroleptics, alcohol, smoking

Table 10.6 Physical causes of sexual dysfunction

Predisposing	Precipitating	Maintaining
Traumatic sexual experience (e.g. sexual abuse)	Childbirth	Anxiety
	Physical illness	Dysfunctional cycle of thoughts and beliefs (e.g. preoccupation with performance or expectation of failure)
'Repressed' upbringing	Mental illness, especially depression	
Cultural/personal attitude towards sex	Medication	
	Alcohol or substance abuse	Relationship conflict
	Sexual trauma	Poor communication with partner
	Stress	Misunderstanding of problem
	Marital/relationship disharmony, including infidelity	

Table 10.7 Predisposing, precipitating and maintaining factors in sexual dysfunction

- **Women:** ask about interest, subjective level of arousal, anxiety about sex, pain on intercourse (when and where), ability to achieve orgasm
- Ask about previous problems
- Obtain a medical history, including medication
- Obtain a psychiatric history and screen for current disorder
- Ask about alcohol and substance use
- Carry out a physical examination and further investigations as required

Management

The management of sexual dysfunction includes:
- thorough assessment, counselling and education
- treatment of any physical causes (if possible) and addressing modifiable risk factors, e.g. smoking, alcohol, medication
- drugs and physical treatments, such as phosphodiesterase–5 (PDE5) inhibitors (e.g. sildenafil (Viagra)), intracavernosal injection of prostaglandin before intercourse and vacuum pumps
- using sex therapy, which is effective in around two-thirds of cases

Learning disability

11.1 Clinical scenario

A change in usual behaviour

Presentation

Philip is a 19-year-old man with a history of severe learning disability (LD) and autism. His mother and carers have observed a change in his behaviour, which they describe as agitated and isolative. They are worried about him and not sure what is wrong.

Diagnostic approach

Assessment needs to take place together with somebody who knows Philip well. His level of understanding, normal behaviour and personality will need to be established. Has a cause for his LD been established? The differential diagnosis is initially very broad and includes psychiatric conditions, such as depression, and physical health problems, such as dysphagia and reflux. More history is needed.

Initial history

Alone, Philip is quiet and withdrawn. It is difficult to establish rapport and he shouts, 'Go away!' Having his mother present allows more progress. He has greasy hair and his mother says that he is not allowing carers to wash him. He is unable to answer questions about mood; however, his mother has noted that he is spending more time alone, no longer watching his favourite TV programmes or finishing his meals, and sleeping poorly. He is also more agitated than usual. These changes have occurred over a period of about six weeks.

Diagnostic approach

Thorough assessment has revealed a number of behaviours indicative of depression. It would be easy to start an antidepressant but if there is depression present, it may have modifiable aetiological factors. He should be asked about recent life events. Reasons for his behaviour should also be considered, e.g. he may not be washing because he is in pain or because he is avoiding abusive carers. Further questioning about physical health and a physical examination are needed.

Further history

His mother reports that, recently, Philip has had two unexplained falls and that, on occasion, he has appeared unresponsive. She thought he was just being stubborn. Physical examination shows some bite marks on his tongue and bruising from the falls. His parents recently separated, and Philip and his mother moved to a new area; this did involve a change in carers, but his mother believes they are very professional and kind.

Diagnostic approach

The history of falls and physical examination are strongly suggestive of seizures. Philip should have further neurological assessment, including an electroencephalogram (EEG) and neuroimaging. LD and epilepsy are commonly comorbid and Philip is likely to require antiepileptic medication, which in itself may resolve the problems.

There have also been several significant life events that should be included in the formulation of predisposing, precipitating and maintaining factors. If possible, Philip should be treated at home to avoid further destabilisation, although an admission could be justified because of frequent seizures and carer respite. Psychological and social interventions should not be neglected. Antidepressants can lower seizure threshold, so simply starting an antidepressant could have made the situation worse. Philip should be kept informed as best as possible and his capacity to take decisions about medication should be considered. A multimodal, multidisciplinary treatment plan is the key to success.

11.2 Learning disability

LD is the preferred term now for the ICD-10 diagnosis 'mental retardation'. In DSM-IV, it is classified as an axis II disorder along with personality disorders. It is important to identify these patients as they are a group at increased need of care and support and have a higher prevalence of behavioural disturbance and psychiatric comorbidity. LD can be subclassified as mild, moderate, severe or profound, as detailed in **Table 11.1**.

There are three components required for a diagnosis:

- low intellectual performance (IQ of 70 or less)
- onset from birth/early childhood
- impairment across a wide range of normal functions

Epidemiology

The epidemiology of LD can be summarised as follows:

- The World Health Organization estimates a prevalence of 3% of the population, with a slight excess in males; mild LD accounts for the bulk of these cases (**Table 11.1**). For example, in the UK, LD affects 1.2 million people; in 210,000 of these, the LD is either severe or profound
- The incidence has fallen in recent years; however, prevalence has remained the same. This is a result of improvements in prevention but a concurrent increase in survival of existing patients

The prevalence of psychiatric disorder in LD is 15–30%. This is around four to five times the normal population prevalence. The prevalence of schizophrenia is estimated to be 3%. There is also an increased risk of affective disorders, anxiety disorders and dementia.

Similarly, physical disability is more common in LD, especially with increasing severity. Sensory dysfunction, motor disorders, poor sphincter control and epilepsy should all be screened for. One-third of those with LD will experience seizures at some point, 15% are unable to walk and 10% are incontinent.

Causes/pathogenesis

The cause of many cases of LD, especially mild LD, is not established and may represent the 'tail end' of normal distribution. Nonetheless, attempting to identify an aetiology is important:

- because there may be a specific treatment, e.g. dietary modification to exclude phenylalanine in phenylketonuria
- to enable predictions regarding the course

Degree of severity	Intelligence quotient (IQ)	Percentage of learning difficulty cases	Prevalence	Description and 'prognosis'	Aetiology
Mild	50–69	85%	2.5%	Mental age: 9–10 Often not obviously distinguishable from normal in early childhood, some delay in meeting developmental milestones. Can usually achieve independence in self-care and practical skills, though this may take longer than normal. Difficulties with academic schoolwork	Tail end of normal distribution ⟶
Moderate	35–49	10%	0.4%	Mental age: 6–8 Slow development of comprehension and use of language. Delayed motor skills and self-care. Limited progress in schoolwork. May be able to do simple work with guidance. Independence rare	
Severe	20–34	3–4%	0.1% (combined)	Mental age: 3–5 Help required with daily tasks and only capable of simple speech	
Profound	<20	1–2%		Mental age: <3 Very disabled in all domains. Severely limited in comprehension, rudimentary non-verbal communication, mobility problems, unable to care for basic needs. Require constant help and supervision	More likely to have identifiable cause

Table 11.1 Subtypes of learning disability

- to identify possible complications early, e.g. cardiovascular malformations in Down's syndrome
- to help the parents, carers and individual come to terms with the condition
- to aid advice regarding risks for future pregnancies

Table 11.2 shows specific causes of LD, which can be subclassified as genetic, intrauterine, perinatal and postnatal. Cases may of course result from an interaction of several factors.

Genetic
Single gene, autosomal dominant disorder, e.g. tuberous sclerosis, neurofibromatosis
Single gene, autosomal recessive disorder, e.g. phenylketonuria
X-linked disorders, e.g. fragile X syndrome, Lesch–Nyhan syndrome
Chromosomal disorder, e.g. Down's syndrome, XYY syndrome
Partial chromosomal deletion, e.g. Prader–Willi syndrome, Cri du chat syndrome

Intrauterine
Intrauterine infections especially rubella, cytomegalovirus, toxoplasmosis, herpes simplex, HIV and syphilis
Folate deficiency
Exposure to teratogens
Fetal alcohol syndrome, smoking/drugs in pregnancy
Hydrocephalus
Complications of pregnancy, e.g. diabetes, antepartum haemorrhage, placental insufficiency, rhesus incompatibility, pre-eclampsia

Perinatal
Prematurity
Brain trauma
Hypoxia
Hyperbilirubinaemia
Infections

Postnatal
Head injury
Infections, e.g. meningitis
Brain tumour
Severe, prolonged seizures
Malnutrition: more common in developing countries (especially iodine, iron and protein deficiency)
Poverty
Neglect and abuse

Table 11.2 Some specific causes of learning disability

Prevention

Measures for prevention include:

- **Genetic counselling** and screening should be offered to those who already have a child with LD or if there is a family history
- **Optimal antenatal care**: involve obstetric care from early in pregnancy with minimisation of exposure to alcohol, smoking and other teratogens. Amniocentesis, chorionic villus sampling and ultrasonography allow early detection of many conditions associated with LD. Termination may be offered
- **Optimal perinatal care**: difficult deliveries (e.g. breech, twins) should be identified promptly and properly managed to reduce trauma, hypoxia and other adverse outcomes. Premature babies should be cared for in a specialised environment
- **Optimal postnatal care**: to include neonatal screening for metabolic disorders such as phenylketonuria, regular checks for sensory problems and developmental delay, and a programme of immunisations against measles, mumps and rubella, and meningitis, among other infectious diseases

Clinical features

LD may be suspected for a wide variety of reasons. It is likely that LD may be picked up prenatally or physical characteristics might arouse doctors' and parents' suspicions shortly after birth:

- Children may present with delayed milestones, academic difficulties, behavioural problems or social difficulties
- Adolescents may present because of social isolation, inappropriate sexual behaviour or evident immaturity
- Adults tend to present with problems relating to everyday activities (e.g. requirement of extra support with forms) or problems with the transition to independent life (e.g. finding employment, marriage, raising children)

As a general rule, difficulties are accentuated during periods of stress.

Psychiatric illness in learning disability

Challenging behaviour is the most common reason for referral in LD (**Table 11.3**). This may represent undiagnosed psychiatric

Nature of behaviour	Examples
Violence to self or others	Hitting, biting, head-banging, scratching, spitting
Socially inappropriate behaviours	Shouting, tantrums, running away, stealing, undressing publicly, urinating in public/in inappropriate places, unsolicited sexual advances
Other	Body rocking, flapping, pica (eating non-edible objects), kleptomania

Table 11.3 Commonly observed 'challenging' behaviours

illness. Making specific diagnoses can be difficult owing to language deficits. Schizophrenia, for example, may present with simple, repetitive hallucinations and persecutory delusions whereas depression may manifest with motor and behavioural changes rather than a verbal expression of low mood or anhedonia.

Clinical insight

Diagnostic overshadowing describes the tendency of clinicians to overlook symptoms of mental (and physical) health problems in patients with learning disability and instead attribute them to being part of 'having an intellectual disability'.

Approach to the patient

The following should be carried out:

- ascertain the level of understanding and ability to communicate
- obtain a collateral history where possible as it is essential to establish normal temperament, changes in observed behaviour and changes in the usual environment
- obtain a developmental history, including details of pregnancy, issues around birth and in early childhood (to consider problems listed in **Table 11.2**)
- assess global functioning and social circumstances
- ask whether there is a family history of learning disability and mental illness
- check for physical and sensory disability
- screen for comorbid psychiatric and medical illness

Investigations

Investigations (when LD is suspected) include:

- thorough physical examination
- biochemical studies
- karyotyping and genetic testing
- neuroimaging
- EEG
- neuropsychological assessment: including IQ testing
- occupational therapy input for functional assessment of activities of daily living

Intelligence quotient

Intelligence should be formally assessed using a standardised test such as the Wechsler Adult Intelligence Scale (WAIS). Different formats are available for children and adults. The score is generally expressed as an 'intelligence quotient' (IQ), which was originally derived from the equation:

$$IQ = \text{mental age/chronological age} \times 100$$

Nowadays, tables are used and the 'average score' for any group should be 100. Intelligence should follow a broadly normal distribution; thus 95% of the population has an IQ between 70 and 130 (±2 standard deviations from the mean). However, the reality is that more people have an IQ below the normal range than above. This excess is attributable to a mixture of genetic and environmental factors (see Causes/pathogenesis).

IQ scores need to be interpreted with care for many reasons ranging from use of non-primary language to mental state at the time of examination, concentration and impact of medication.

Diagnostic criteria and differential diagnoses

For diagnostic criteria between degrees of LD, see **Table 11.1**.
Otherwise, the differential diagnoses include:

- below average IQ but with IQ>70
- autism/autistic spectrum disorder (see **Chapter 12**)
- acquired brain injury
- severe and enduring psychiatric illness

- severe neglect

Management

Many will not require any specific service provision, and psychiatric problems can be managed by general psychiatric services should they arise.

Among those who do require additional support, the nature of this will be determined by their overall level of functioning, problems in specific domains (e.g. communication or activities of daily living), physical health problems (e.g. epilepsy), concurrent psychiatric disorder, challenging behaviours and level of family support. Consequently, a multidisciplinary approach with psychiatrists, paediatricians, neurologists, occupational therapists, speech and language therapists, nurses, educational support and social support is the norm depending on the needs of the patient.

General treatment points

These include:

- psychoeducation and support for the family/carers is critical
- set realistic goals and highlight potential difficulties
- educational support including 'statementing'
- optimise sensory problems with hearing and visual aids
- challenging behaviour should be managed with behavioural therapy and environmental modification in the first instance
- medication should be used cautiously owing to an increased incidence of side-effects; the need for psychotropic medication should be reviewed regularly
- treat comorbid medical and psychiatric problems and be aware that these will present in different ways, e.g. depression with behavioural change rather than expressed low mood; use of specialist guidelines such as the DC-LD diagnostic criteria for use with adults with learning disabilities, may aid accurate diagnosis
- historically, the medicalisation of LD led to institutional care of patients with LD; the subsequent isolation and occasional abuse of patients brought about huge changes in care provision, including the concept of 'normalisation', which holds

that optimal care does not necessarily mean segregation from the rest of society but that a physical environment and living routine should be implemented that are as normal as possible

- although the trend over the past few decades has been away from institutionalised care, hospitals may provide respite, assessment or treatment for comorbid conditions
- consider the well-being of the family/carers and what impact their not being available might have
- beware of increased risk of physical, emotional and sexual abuse

Complications/prognosis

LD is a lifelong condition of variable impact. As expected, there is a reduced life expectancy, depending on the aetiology of the disability.

The presence of a learning disability is associated with:

- epilepsy (~30%)
- autism (up to 30%)
- structural brain damage
- visual and/or hearing impairment
- increased frequency of physical health problems
- communication difficulties
- poor coping strategies and vulnerability to exploitation
- stigmatisation
- adverse life events
- adverse living environment
- family difficulties
- challenging behaviours (**Table 11.3**)

Child and adolescent psychiatry

12.1 Clinical scenario

An overly active boy

Presentation

George is an 8-year-old boy referred by his GP to an child psychiatrist. The primary school teacher prompted his parents to seek advice and she has provided a note saying "

> …he's incredibly difficult to manage in the classroom, always talking, always getting out of his chair, never able to finish any work and constantly getting in trouble. Just last week he saw a power socket in the classroom with a loose screw and ended up sticking a pencil inside and almost electrocuting himself!

Diagnostic approach

In children it is common for behaviour rather than psychiatric symptoms to lead to presentation. More history is needed (**Table 12.4**). Key to this will be talking with the parents and whether they share the teacher's concerns. Generally, teachers are an excellent resource as they have a wide experience of what is normal. Sometimes, it could just be an issue with the teacher or school environment. The differential diagnosis is wide with emotional, behavioural and developmental conditions all meriting consideration.

Initial history

George is brought to the appointment by his parents. They divorced 2 years ago, but both attend. His mother says that George's behaviour has been getting worse over the last few years. There is a slightly hostile atmosphere in the room. She had a normal pregnancy with George, but smoked

	Motor skills	Vision and fine movement	Hearing and language	Social behaviour
Newborn	Symmetrical movements, limbs flexed	Looks at light/faces in direct line of vision	Response to noises/voices	Responds to parents
Supine infant (2–3 months)	Raises head in prone position, loses grasp reflex	Tracks objects	Cries, coos, grunts	Squeals with pleasure appropriately Smiles discriminately
Sitting infant (6–9 months)	~6/12: sits erect with support ~9/12: sits unsupported	6/12: 'palmar' grasp 7/12: transfers objects between hands 9/12: looks for dropped toys; develops pincer grip	Babbles Localises sound 45 cm lateral to either ear	Develops stranger shyness and separation anxiety Plays 'peak-a-boo'
Toddler (18–24 months)	12/12: stands unsupported but briefly and makes first steps 24/12: climbs stairs	12/12: drops toys and watches where they go 16/12: uses spoon or fork	12/12: vocabulary of 1–3 words 24/12: vocabulary of >200 words; makes phrases	Waves goodbye, cooperates with dressing Is prone to temper tantrums 24/12: dry by day
Communi-cating child (3–4 years)	Stands on one leg Jumps Pedals on bike	Mature pencil grip Draws a circle and a cross	Makes complete sentences	Plays cooperatively with other children Imitates parents Attends to own toileting needs Questions everything

. Adapted from Burton N, 2009 Clinical Skills for OSCEs, 3rd edn Oxford : Scion Publishing

Table 12.1 Developmental milestones

throughout. He met his developmental milestones but is not doing well with schoolwork. His mother says that he was a good boy until the age of 5, unlike his brother, who is older and constantly in trouble.

George manages to sit for 15 minutes but is constantly fidgeting, before asking to go to the toilet. When he returns he interrupts the conversation constantly. The specialist nurse takes him out to play in the art room.

Diagnostic approach

This information would indicate a diagnosis of attention deficit and hyperactivity disorder (ADHD; see below) and this should be the working diagnosis. The divorce of the parents and subsequent family dynamics may also play some role and merit further exploration. To obtain some objective information the parents and school are asked to complete a questionnaire. George's parents are given literature about ADHD and told that the specialist nurse will visit to discuss the condition and possible behavioural strategies.

Given his difficulties with schoolwork, neuropsychological testing is requested. This is used much more in children. George scores 90, but the psychologist says his poor concentration probably lowered the true score. Nonetheless, this excludes the possibility of learning disability.

An educational psychologist visits school and encourages a less punitive teaching approach. Strategies to minimise distracting environmental factors have an initial positive response.

> ### Clinical insight
>
> In child psychiatry, education, support, behavioural and environmental interventions and active monitoring by multiple agencies are generally used first rather than medication.

Further history

Three months later the family return. The mother has attended a parent training programme and tried to improve the family's diet, but it has made little difference. The Conners questionnaires have been completed by George's parents and school and are strongly supportive of the diagnosis.

Diagnostic approach

There has now been adequate time for comprehensive multidisciplinary assessment and a variety of psychosocial interventions. Assuming there are no contraindications, a trial of medication is indicated to reduce symptoms and to prevent deterioration and further problems. Side-effects need to be discussed, which in this case would include abdominal pain, nausea and vomiting, and growth suppression in the longer term. Regular follow-up is arranged and, despite some initial reservations on the part of his father, George responds extremely well to the medication.

12.2 Overview of child psychiatry

> The childhood shows the man
> As morning shows the day.
>
> John Milton 1608–1674,
> *Paradise Regained*

Children are referred to child psychiatrists by parents or teachers because of concern about behaviour, emotional state or development. Signs and symptoms of mental disorder are common in children and adolescents and the art of child psychiatry lies in deciding what is on the spectrum of normal experience and what constitutes a psychiatric disorder. For example, although temper tantrums are a normal phenomenon when aged two, they cease to be so when aged 11 or 12.

Childhood is a period of rapid physical and psychological development and problems need to be judged in their developmental context. **Table 12.1** outlines important early developmental milestones.

Epidemiology

Table 12.2 shows the epidemiology of common childhood disorders.

Disorder	Prevalence (%)	Male–female ratio
Attention deficit and hyperactivity disorder	1–2%	3:1

Anxiety disorders
    Separation anxiety
    Simple phobia
    Obsessive–compulsive disorder
	0.7–12.0%
	2.4–3.6%
	1.9%
		Female > male

Autism	0.1–0.6%	3:1
Conduct disorder	>4%	3:1
Depression	1–5% (rising with age)	Starts equal, becoming female excess post puberty

Eating disorders
    Anorexia nervosa
    Bulimia nervosa
	0.36–0.83% (girls only)
	1.5
		1:10
		1:8

Elimination disorders Enuresis	10% at 5 years; 1% at 15 years	1:1 at 5 years; 2:1 at 15 years
School refusal	0.7%	1:1
Tourette's disorder	0.05%	Male excess

Table 12.2 Epidemiology of common and important childhood disorders

Preschool children

In preschool children, the prevalence of moderate to severe behavioural and emotional problems is 7%, with boys affected more than girls. The prevalence of mild behavioural and emotional problems is 15%. These disorders are associated with maternal depression, marital conflict, delayed development of language and large family size.

Middle childhood

In middle childhood (10–11 years old), the point prevalence of child psychiatric disorder is 6.8%. This can be up to twofold greater in urban areas. Conduct disorder is the most common diagnosis (~3/5), followed by emotional disorders (~2/5). Children with chronic illness have double the rate of psychiatric illness (11%) and children with epilepsy have a rate approaching 35%.

Adolescence

In adolescence, the prevalence of psychiatric disorder increases to around 9%. The male–female ratio is 1:1.5. Depressive symptomatology increases after puberty, with 40% of teenagers reporting misery and depression, 20% negative self-perception and 7% suicidal feelings.

Causes

The aetiology of childhood psychiatric disorders is complex and usually multifactorial. Its development depends not just on the presence and interaction of risk factors but also on the presence or otherwise of protective factors. **Table 12.3** outlines some aetiological factors to consider.

Approach to the patient

General principles are as follows:

- Spend time establishing rapport with the child and family
- Topics for exploration are detailed in **Table 12.4**; unlike adult psychiatry, history may be obtained predominantly from the parent or carer
- Flexibility in assessment is paramount, but optimally there are three core components to the history-taking process:
  1. **Family interview**: perhaps the most important component as it gives a sense of what the problem is. This provides a good opportunity to construct a genogram and observe the family dynamic
  2. **Child interview**: may or may not be performed alone; it is important to assess the child's perception of the 'problem'. Remember to use open-ended questions. This may be the best opportunity to observe play

Domains	Risk factors	Protective factors
Constitutional factors	Genetic	Above-average IQ
	Chromosomal abnormalities	
	Low IQ	
Physical factors	Intrauterine infections	Meeting developmental milestones
	Prematurity	
	Injury, especially brain damage	
Temperamental factors	Irregularity	Positive temperament
	Negative moods	Sociable
	Poor adaptability	High self-esteem
Family factors	Family conflict	Close-knit family
	Separation and divorce of parents	Clear roles
	Domestic violence	Good relationships
	Adverse parenting (e.g. rejection, inconsistency, punitiveness, failure to set rules, failure to monitor)	
	Parental criminality	
Environmental and social factors	Stressful life events	Supportive friendship
	Poor schooling	Ongoing education
	Low socioeconomic class	

Table 12.3 Aetiological factors in child and adolescent psychiatric disorders

3. **Collateral history** from school and other agencies: this is often critical to the diagnostic process

Investigations
Use questionnaires and specific rating scales, e.g. Conners Rating Scale in ADHD. Also consider psychometric testing.

Assessment component	Specifics
Demographic details	
Presenting problem	Frequency Severity Onset Duration Exacerbating/relieving factors Carer/child explanation
Other problems or complaints	General health (e.g. seizures, sleeping, eating) Interests, activities, hobbies Relationship with family and peers Prevailing mood Temperament and behaviour Level of functioning: attention span
Recent life events	–
Family	Parent/sibling mental and physical health, personality Quality of parenting Problems at home Relationship with family members (e.g. degree of affection, openness) Genogram
School record	Attendance, educational attainment
Personal history	Pregnancy and delivery Mother–child relationship Developmental milestones (**Table 12.1**)
Observation of child	Appearance: evidence of neglect or injury; nutritional status Interactions with interviewer and family members (eye contact, spontaneous talk, shyness, etc.) Level of activity, including involuntary movements Attention and concentration Mood and range of emotions expressed Habits and mannerisms Delusions, hallucinations, thought disorder
Observation of family	Pattern of interaction (e.g. arguments, shouting) Communication Emotional atmosphere (concern, criticism, tension, etc.)
Physical examination	–

Table 12.4 Components of an assessment in child psychiatry

Diagnostic criteria

Disorders in child psychiatry can be grouped into three broad categories (**Table 12.5**). These are emotional disorders, behavioural disorders and developmental disorders. In reality, the dividing line between the three groups is not always clear. ADHD can, for example, be classified under behavioural disorders or as a developmental disorder (of attention and activity).

Clinical insight

A full clinical assessment in child psychiatry can take a great deal of time, especially when observation, physical examination and collateral history are included. Do not feel the need to fit everything into one interview. More than one assessment is often required, and may be preferable.

Category	Disorders
Emotional disorders	Anxiety disorders Phobias Depression Obsessive–compulsive disorder Somatisation disorders Deliberate self-harm
Behavioural disorders	Conduct disorder Oppositional defiant disorder Attention deficit and hyperactivity disorder School refusal
Developmental disorders	Learning difficulties Autism Asperger's syndrome Tourette's syndrome
Other problems affecting children	Enuresis Encopresis Eating disorders Child abuse Psychosis Post-traumatic stress disorder

Table 12.5 Categorisation of childhood disorders

Another difference in child psychiatry is the greater use of multiaxial diagnosis (**Table 12.6**).

For detailed diagnostic criteria on individual conditions, see below.

12.3 Developmental disorders

Developmental disorders include learning disability, autism and Asperger's syndrome.

12.4 Learning disability

See **Chapter 11**.

12.5 Autism

First described by Leo Kanner in 1943, autism is a pervasive developmental disorder characterised by a core triad of difficulties:

1. **Communication**: there is delayed or total lack of language acquisition in both expression and comprehension. Conversation is not initiated or sustained. Language (if used) may be stereotyped or repetitive with, for example, repetition of set phrases, use of neologisms or pronominal reversal
2. **Social development**: there are abnormalities in reciprocal social interaction. This may present as disinterest in other people ('autistic aloneness'), manifest in childhood as not seeking comfort, solitary play or paucity of interaction with peers. There may be limited eye contact, facial expression or use of gestures such as pointing or showing

Axis I	Psychiatric diagnosis (ICD-10), e.g. depression
Axis II	Specific developmental disorder, e.g. autism
Axis III	Intelligence, e.g. borderline learning disability
Axis IV	Medical conditions, e.g. epilepsy
Axis V	Psychosocial circumstances, e.g. foster care
Axis VI	Level of functioning, e.g. moderate social disability

Table 12.6 The ICD-10 multiaxial system for childhood disorders

3. Autism is characterised by a restricted, repetitive and stereo-typed pattern of behaviour, interests and activities. Patients may also lack imaginative play and dislike changes in routine

Epidemiology

The prevalence is approximately 1 in 1000, rising to 6 in 1000 for autistic spectrum disorder. The male–female ratio is 3:1. Unlike many childhood disorders, the prevalence is evenly distributed between socioeconomic groups.

Causes

The aetiology is currently thought to be related to an interplay of organic factors, especially genetic loading and obstetric and environmental risk factors. Certain genetic conditions, such as tuberous sclerosis and fragile X syndrome, have very high rates of comorbid autism.

Clinical features

Table 12.7 shows some of the more common reasons for presentation.

- the onset of these problems needs to be before the patient is 36 months old, although diagnosis usually occurs some years later
- autism is highly comorbid with learning disability, with 50% having an intelligence quotient (IQ) <50 and 95% <100. Verbal IQ is lower than non-verbal IQ. Epilepsy is also common, with 25% having seizures

Differential diagnoses

These include:

- learning disability without autism
- Asperger's syndrome (see below)
- deafness
- psychosocial deprivation
- certain rare disorders, e.g. Rett's syndrome, disintegrative psychosis

Cannot be comforted when upset
Little interest or response to cuddling
No exploratory play
Repetitive, obsessional play with just 1 or 2 toys
Difficulty expressing needs
Inappropriate laughing/ giggling
Echoing of words or phrases
Spinning of objects or self
Delayed (or not met) developmental milestones
Insisting that things are kept the same
Lack of fear of danger
Tantrums
Paucity of friendship
Struggling educationally
An overall sense that they 'different'

Table 12.7 Some common presenting problems in autism (usually expressed by parents or teachers)

Management

There is no specific treatment for autism. After thorough neuropsychological evaluation and identification of specific problems, treatment centres on parental support and education, optimisation of the educational environment (e.g. provision of a teaching assistant), behavioural modification (e.g. using the LOVAAS technique of applied behaviour analysis) and treatment of associated medical and psychiatric conditions. Low-dose antipsychotics are sometimes used to reduce problem behaviours.

Prognosis

Only 5–10% gain full independence. Poor prognostic indicators include low IQ and lack of language.

12.6 Asperger's syndrome

Asperger's syndrome is a pervasive developmental disorder generally considered to be part of the autistic spectrum. It is characterised by the same abnormalities in social interaction and a restricted, stereotyped, repetitive range of interests and activities, as seen in autism.

Unlike autism, there is no general delay in language or cognitive development. IQ is in the normal (and sometimes high) range. The exact prevalence is difficult to ascertain, but there is a male–female ratio of 8:1.

> **Clinical insight**
>
> **Asperger's syndrome** is named after the Austrian paediatrician Hans Asperger (1906–1980), who first described the condition and referred to his patients as 'my little professors'.

Management

Treatment (if required) centres on general advice, optimising education provision and support with social skills training. It is a lifelong condition, but the prognosis is much better than for autism and individuals are generally independent and sometimes extremely successful.

12.7 Behavioural disorders

Behavioural disorders include hyperkinetic disorders, conduct disorder and school refusal.

12.8 Hyperkinetic disorders/attention deficit and hyperactivity disorder

ADHD, or 'hyperkinetic disorder' as it is referred to in ICD-10, is characterised by the three core symptoms of:

1. inattention
2. hyperactivity
3. impulsivity

It is a diagnosis that has been the subject of vigorous debate and some controversy, not least because of a prevalence rate of 7.5% if DSM-IV criteria are used. Point prevalence according to ICD-10 criteria is 1–2%, with a male–female ratio of 3:1.

Although there has been criticism that ADHD is simply a label for active, creative but difficult to manage children, there is a great deal of evidence to suggest that a child meeting the criteria for ADHD is prone to reduced academic achievement, increased risk of accidents, low self-esteem, sleep problems and peer relationship issues in the short term, and reduced employment success, increased criminal activity and development of other psychiatric disorders in the longer term.

Clinical features

Inattention

Children with ADHD are noticeably distractible and find it difficult to concentrate. They may have a propensity to shift chaotically between activities and fail to finish tasks. Parents and teachers may also note them to be careless with details, disorganised, forgetful and unable to engage in tasks requiring sustained attention.

Hyperactivity

The child will be noticeably energetic, may fidget with hands and feet, have a tendency to explore new environments while running, jumping, climbing and often making a great deal of noise.

Impulsivity

The child may be noted to be unable to wait his turn, talk excessively and interrupt others or blurt out answers in class. More risky behaviour may be seen in terms of poor road safety and generally being accident prone.

These symptoms should be present at developmentally inappropriate levels, start **before the age of 7,** be present across two or more settings and be persistent over time.

Differential diagnoses

These include:

- conduct disorder
- depression/anxiety
- mania (rare)

Management

General

Psychoeducation for parents, family and school teachers. Family therapy may be considered in some cases.

Behavioural interventions

These focus on assessment of problem behaviours at home and school, and instigation of a strategy of positive reinforcement and negative feedback for unacceptable behaviours. Caregivers will be encouraged to maintain clear and consistent boundaries, break down tasks into manageable chunks and create environments with fewer distractions.

Medication

This is one disorder in child psychiatry in which medication is regularly used. The currently available drugs attenuate core symptoms but do not 'cure' per se. Medication should only be initiated by specialists and requires careful monitoring. The response rate is good, with 70% of children showing improvement. Psychostimulants such as methylphenidate (e.g. Ritalin) and dexamfetamine are used. Common and potentially problematic side-effects of these include insomnia, anorexia and growth reduction. Other drugs used include atomoxetine, which is a noradrenaline reuptake inhibitor, and, rarely, clonidine.

Other

Other popular but less evidence-based interventions include dietary modification, such as the addition of omega-3, or elimination of artificial flavours, colours, sweeteners and preservatives (Feingold diet).

12.9 Conduct disorder

Conduct disorder (CD) is a behavioural syndrome characterised by a persistent pattern of antisocial aggressive or defiant behaviour, which, at its most extreme, amounts to a major violation of age-appropriate social expectations. It is therefore much more severe than ordinary childish mischief or rebelliousness. Severe aggression, stealing, lying, destructiveness and even pyromania may be present. Commonly, relationship difficulties are also present.

ICD-10 divides CD into **socialised CD**, in which the child has a peer group who often also act in this way, and **unsocialised CD**, in which the child is rejected by peers and acts alone. **Oppositional defiant disorder** (ODD) is a type of conduct disorder seen in younger children in whom the more severe dissocial or aggressive acts are absent.

Epidemiology

CD has a point prevalence of 4% in 10- to 11-year-olds, making it the most common psychiatric disorder in older children and teenagers. This has been found to be significantly higher in inner city cohorts. There is a large male preponderance.

Clinical features

There are different manifestations at different ages, e.g. temper tantrums in early childhood or truancy in older children. The duration of problems must be longer than 6 months. Typically, these include:

- temper tantrums
- severe arguments
- disobedience
- blaming of others for own mistakes
- violence to people, property or animals
- bullying
- police record
- inappropriate sexual behaviour

Differential diagnoses

There is significant overlap with hyperkinetic disorders and emotional disorders. If the criteria for hyperkinetic disorder are met, this takes precedence. If the criteria for emotional disorders are met, a diagnosis of mixed disorder of conduct and emotions can be made.

Management

Management centres initially on thorough assessment of the behaviour and exclusion of other psychiatric conditions. Psychotherapy, including family therapy, problem-solving therapy and behavioural therapy, may help, along with parenting skills training.

Prognosis
Of those with CD, 50% go on to develop dissocial personality disorder. Substance abuse, domestic violence and criminality are common.

12.10 School refusal

This is the refusal to attend or remain at school. It is important to differentiate school refusal from truancy. Unlike school refusal, truancy is intended, often accompanied by other antisocial behaviours, likely to be associated with poor academic performance and with a family history of antisocial behaviour.

School refusal is relatively common, accounting for approximately 5% of referrals and affects males and females in equal proportion. There are three main incidence peaks with differing aetiological factors:

- **5-year-olds**: due to separation anxiety
- **11-year-olds**: most common and often due to the transition from primary to secondary school
- **14- to 16-year-olds**: a symptom of psychiatric disorder, usually depression or phobia (particularly social phobia)

Management
Management involves identifying underlying reasons. If the presentation is acute then a return to school should be facilitated as soon as possible. If it is chronic, a graded return is often preferable. Any specific disorders, e.g. social phobia, should be treated. Younger children have a better prognosis. School refusal is associated with later development of mood, anxiety and other neurotic disorders.

12.11 Emotional disorders

Emotional disorders include anxiety disorders, depression, obsessive–compulsive disorder and self-harm and suicide.

12.12 Anxiety disorders

Separation anxiety disorder (see also **Chapter 7**) of childhood is a severe, persistent fear of separation in children. Children are clingy and fear that any separation may be permanent and that harm may befall them or their attachment figure should they be separated. It is frequently associated with nightmares, mild physical symptoms and school refusal. The condition is often related to some sort of stressful event (e.g. the loss of a pet) and parents may be overprotective. Management is through careful identification of precipitants, parental education and managed separation.

12.13 Depression

Diagnosis is made using the same criteria as in adults, but there may be differences in presentation:
- apathy, failure to thrive, tantrums, regressive behaviour in younger children
- somatisation, school refusal, sleep problems in older children
  See also **Chapter 4.**

Epidemiology

The prevalence increases with age. Less than 1–2% of children are affected when prepubertal, rising to 3–5% in adolescents. The sex ratio starts equally but becomes skewed to a female excess. Self-harm is relatively common in this age group; therefore, treatment of depression is important.

Management

After 'watchful waiting', psychotherapy is usually first-line treatment, usually in the form of cognitive–behavioural therapy, interpersonal therapy or family therapy. Medication is used with caution, in part because of a potential increase in suicidal ideation as a side-effect. Fluoxetine is the only licensed antidepressant in children.

Prognosis

The younger the age at first presentation, the greater the likelihood of recurrence and the worse the prognosis.

12.14 Obsessive–compulsive disorder

Subclinical obsessions and compulsions are common, occurring in up to 20% of children. Obsessive–compulsive disorder (OCD) commonly starts in adolescence, with presentation and management as in adults (see **Chapter 7**).

12.15 Self-harm and suicide

See **Chapter 5**.

12.16 Other disorders

Other disorders consist of enuresis, encopresis, and tics and Tourette's syndrome.

12.17 Enuresis

A practical definition for enuresis is the involuntary passage of urine after the age at which bladder control is expected. It causes a great deal of distress to parents and children, affects self-esteem and can precipitate bullying and non-participation.

Enuresis can be:
- **primary**: toilet training never achieved. This is usually due to delayed development of the nervous system. Other developmental milestones are often also delayed
- **secondary**: bladder control achieved for at least 6 months and then lost
- **nocturnal** (bed-wetting), which is more common in boys
- **diurnal** (daytime), which is more common in girls

At 5 years old, 10% are affected (male–female ratio 1:1). At 15 years old, 1% are affected (male–female ratio 2:1).

Perhaps surprisingly, around 70% have a family history.

Management

Management is as follows:
- screen for organic causes such as epilepsy, diabetes, urinary tract infection and urinary tract malformation. Refer to paediatricians if any uncertainty

- reassure and provide practical advice, e.g. restricting fluids before bed
- behavioural treatments are very effective and include the use of a star chart to provide positive reinforcement and the 'bell and pad' system (an enuresis alarm which wakes the child on detecting moisture, thereby teaching voiding)
- medication is now rarely used but desmopressin (synthetic antidiuretic hormone) and tricyclic antidepressants (e.g. imipramine) are occasionally helpful

Prognosis is excellent.

12.18 Encopresis

This is the repeated voluntary or involuntary passage of faeces. Encopresis is diagnosed if soiling occurs more than once a month over the age of 4. As with enuresis, it can be divided into primary and secondary causes. Retentive encopresis, which accounts for the vast majority of cases, develops as a consequence of chronic constipation with resulting overflow incontinence. The cause of constipation needs to be established. Both organic (anal fissures, poor diet, Hirschsprung's disease, etc.) and psychological (toileting fears, fear of painful defaecation, etc.) factors ought to be considered.

Management

Management involves destigmatisation of the problem, lifestyle changes, behavioural approaches (e.g. star charts) and the use of laxatives or stool softeners. The prognosis is good, with >85% of cases resolving within a year.

12.19 Tics and Tourette's syndrome

Tics are rapid, involuntary, repetitive, purposeless motor movements or vocalisations.

Simple tics

These can be motor or vocal. Examples include blinking eyes, shrugging shoulders, grimacing and grunting, or throat clearing.

Complex motor tics

Complex motor tics may include jumping and hitting oneself, whereas complex vocal tics include repeating what others say (echolalia) or shouting obscenities (coprolalia). Tic frequency is exacerbated by stress. Tics can be suppressed voluntarily, although this may lead to a build up of tension and possibly a burst of tics.

ICD-10 subdivides tics into:

- transient tic disorder: motor or vocal tics lasting less than 12 months
- chronic motor or vocal tic disorder: motor or vocal tics lasting more than 12 months
- Tourette's syndrome: vocal **and** multiple motor tics lasting more than 12 months

Epidemiology

Tics affect up to 10% of children up to the age of 10, and are approximately three times more common in boys.

> ### Clinical insight
>
> The public perception of Tourette's syndrome is of people shouting expletives (coprolalia). Although dramatic, coprolalia occurs in only 30% of cases.

Cause

The exact cause of Tourette's syndrome is unknown, but it is a highly heritable disorder involving dysfunction of the basal ganglia, thalamus and frontal cortex. Conditions associated with Tourette's syndrome include OCD, which is comorbid in 30–60% of cases, and ADHD, which is present in over 25%.

Management

Education

Treatment centres initially on education of the patient, family and school about the disorder and, in particular, making sure the child is not punished. Relaxation techniques may also be of benefit in stress-associated tics.

Medication

Pharmacological treatments include antipsychotics, such as risperidone, haloperidol and sulpiride, the α_2-agonist clonidine and certain antidepressants. Psychostimulants prescribed for the treatment of ADHD may exacerbate tics.

Prognosis

The prognosis is good and, although tics can wax and wane or change in nature, they generally decrease in early adulthood.

chapter 13

Mental health services and legislation

The principles of mental health practice are applicable world-wide, but the provision of mental health services varies from one country to another. Differences in funding models contribute to these variations, as does the historical development of the services within a region. Uniquely, compared with other medical specialties, in mental health a significant body of legislation also influences the frameworks and settings in which care is given.

In a book of this size, it would be impossible to review the mental health services and legislation of all its readers' nations. Instead, we use the current framework in England and Wales to illustrate the issues relating to service provision and the key aspects covered by legislation. We hope that readers everywhere will find these examples useful.

13.1 The structure of mental health services

Psychiatric illness is common

As an example, community surveys in the UK indicate that 25% of the population experience significant mental health problems at some point between the ages of 18 and 65. The most common problems are depression and anxiety. The male–female ratio for psychiatric morbidity is approximately 1:1.5. In older people, the prevalence increases, owing in part to the risk of dementia. Psychiatric illness is also highly concentrated in certain groups. For example, just 10% of prisoners have no mental disorder.

Most patients are managed in primary care

Unsurprisingly, 25% of GP consultations (in the UK) relate to mental health problems. The most common presentations in primary care are depression, anxiety and somatisation disorder, but it is estimated that up to 30% of significant illness is missed. **Table 13.1** considers why this may be the case.

Just 15% of detected cases will be referred on to secondary care, which may reflect GPs' confidence in managing mental illness, reluctance on the part of the patient to be referred on, inadequate provision of secondary psychiatric services or simply the low-grade, transient nature of certain problems.

Table 13.2 outlines common features precipitating referral to secondary psychiatric services.

Psychiatric subspecialties

Psychiatry is divided into several specialties and subspecialties
- general adult psychiatry
- old age psychiatry (psychogeriatrics)
- child and adolescent psychiatry
- forensic psychiatry
- eating disorders
- substance misuse services
- liaison psychiatry
- psychotherapy
- neuropsychiatry

Factor	Reason
Patient	Stigma of mental illness
	Cultural issues
	Perception that it is not really a problem or is 'untreatable'
	Reporting only of somatic symptoms
	Concealment of psychosocial stressors and emotions
Doctor	Failure to consider the possibility of mental illness
	Inability to elicit psychiatric symptoms
Circumstantial	Lack of time
	Lack of privacy
	Focus on medical disease

Table 13.1 Why psychiatric diagnoses are missed

Factor	Further information
Diagnosis	Psychosis Treatment-resistant depression or anxiety Dementia Obsessive–compulsive disorder Severe personality disorder Specialist situations, e.g. disorders in childhood or eating disorders
Risk	Suicide attempts or persistent ideation Self-harm Self-neglect Violence
Social circumstances	Inability to function adequately in society because of a mental disorder
Comorbidity	Mental illness in the context of substance misuse, personality disorder, learning disability or physical illness

Table 13.2 Factors typically prompting a referral to secondary mental health services

13.2 The history of psychiatric care

The eighteenth century saw the beginnings of organised mental healthcare in the UK. This came through the opening of an array of asylums, madhouses and lunatic hospitals. These institutions tended to use ineffective physical remedies and mechanical restraint, and it was not until the opening of William Tuke's Retreat in York that a regimen of kindness and compassionate care (so-called 'moral treatment') was introduced.

The number of mental health hospital beds peaked in 1954, after which a change in direction towards community care took place. The emergence of new medical treatments, changing public attitudes to mental illness and a series of abuse scandals probably lie at the heart of this shift.

Table 13.3 outlines some of the advantages and disadvantages of community care. For ways in which patients may access mental healthcare services, see **Figure 13.1**.

Advantages	Disadvantages
Reduced stigmatisation of mental illness Decreases isolation Decreases institutionalisation Generally thought to be cheaper Focus on personal strengths rather than illness	Greater burden on carers Greater burden on mental health staff Limited resources Threat to patient safety Possible increased threat to community safety May paradoxically increase isolation May be failing those most in need (homeless, lacking own social support or non-engaging)

Table 13.3 Advantages and disadvantages of community care

13.3 Structure of mental health services

General practice and emergency departments

GPs see a very different profile of psychiatric disorder from that seen by psychiatrists. The majority of patients will have low-grade neurotic disorders rather than the more severe and enduring psychoses. However, GPs are responsible for identifying those at need of specialist input and referring appropriately.

In contrast, in emergency departments a great deal of deliberate self-harm but also substance misuse, delirium and somatoform disorders are seen.

Community mental health team and multidisciplinary team

The community mental health team (CMHT) is at the centre of mental healthcare provision. It consists of a multidisciplinary team (**Table 13.4**) that covers a set geographical area. If patients are considered to have a severe mental disorder or the complexity of their problems is beyond the capacity of primary healthcare services, they are referred to the CMHT. Referral is followed by initial assessment and, if deemed appropriate, ongoing treatment and support. Assistance will be given in addressing all aetiological factors, which may include:

- specific mental illnesses
- emotional problems

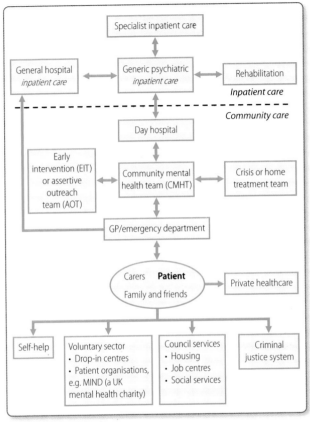

Figure 13.1 Ways in which patients can access mental healthcare services in the UK

- relationship problems
- housing
- medication
- finances and benefits
- employment
- low self-esteem

General adult CMHTs care for those aged 18–65, whereas older adult CMHTs exist for those aged over 65, child and adolescent

Member	Role within the team
Psychiatrist	Medical leadership Education Formulation and diagnosis Prescription of medication Use of legislation Medicolegal responsibility Liaison with other medical specialties
Community psychiatric nurse (CPN)	Co-ordination of care High-frequency patient contact Monitoring of progress/problems Initial assessments Administration of medication Practical advice and support
Social worker	Co-ordination of care Expert help with finances, housing, employment and other entitlements May have further training to become an approved mental health practitioner responsible for co-ordinating Mental Health Act applications
Occupational therapist (OT)	Assessment of skills, disability, living environment Optimisation of environment Promote independence, confidence and self-esteem
Clinical psychologist	Psychological assessment and formulation Specialist testing, e.g. IQ Delivery of talking treatments
Pharmacist	Expert advice on medication, e.g. drug interactions, side-effects, special situations such as pregnancy
Administrative staff	Practical details of running the team Interface between patients and team

Table 13.4 Members of the multidisciplinary team and respective roles

CMHTs for those aged under 18 and learning disability CMHTs for those with learning disability.

Crisis and home treatment teams

Open 24 hours a day, 365 days a year, crisis teams can be considered the emergency departments of psychiatry. They provide prompt assessment, treatment and support to patients in crisis. Work includes being the out-of-hours point of contact and liaison work assessing patients in hospital emergency departments.

Referrals for more intensive monitoring and support come from CMHTs, and the crisis and home treatment teams play a role in determining whether admission to hospital can be avoided. If so, they may undertake home visits up to three times a day, monitoring the response to interventions. The typical multidisciplinary team structure is used, although with a weighting towards community psychiatric nurses.

Assertive outreach team

Often, people with severe mental disorders are reluctant to seek help or engage with treatment. They may appear only at times of crisis, such as when self-harming or causing a public disturbance. The assertive outreach team (AOT) is tasked with engaging these complex patients in treatment, preventing relapse and supporting them in the community.

Early intervention team

The longer an episode of psychosis goes untreated, the poorer the prognosis. The early intervention team (EIT; sometimes also called the early intervention service) aims to improve outcomes by prevention, early detection and intensive intervention in the early stages of psychotic illness.

Day hospital and inpatient units

As the number of psychiatric beds has fallen, the threshold for admission has risen. Although the majority are still admitted informally on a voluntary basis, an increasing proportion of patients are brought in only if acutely disturbed, psychotic or detained under the Mental Health Act. Nonetheless, inpatient care remains an important part of patient management.

Most psychiatric specialties have their own inpatient facilities, and patients should be treated in the most appropriate setting, e.g. those with dementia in a specialist older adult unit.

13.4 Rehabilitation

This may be required following long periods of inpatient treatment as an intermediate step to reintegration into the community. During this time, psychosocial aspects of care may be comprehensively assessed and addressed.

13.5 Care programme approach

Once a patient is being treated by secondary psychiatric services, their care is managed using the **care programme approach (CPA)**. The aim of this is to standardise the planning and provision of care. The care programme approach has four 'cornerstones':

1. **assessment**: this should cover psychiatric, medical and social needs as well as assessing risk
2. **a care plan**: the formulation of a written care plan that addresses the identified health and social care needs. It should include early indicators of relapse and planning for what to do in periods of crisis
3. **a care co-ordinator**: the appointment of a care co-ordinator (previously called a key worker) to keep in close touch with the patient and to monitor their care
4. **regular review**: this should occur at least every 6 months, ideally including everybody participating in a patient's care. Agreed changes are then made to the care plan

13.6 Legislation

The Mental Health Act

Severe mental illness can sometimes cause patients to be at risk of harm to themselves or others. When they lack insight into this, and consequently refuse appropriate management, they may require detention and treatment against their will.

The **Mental Health Act** of 1983 (updated in 2007) provides the legal framework in England and Wales for managing this necessary balance between the rights of the individual and the rights of society. Key sections of the Mental Health Act are shown in **Table 13.5**.

Section and role	Details	Maximum duration	Application and potential outcomes
136 Police emergency power Allows police to remove a person to a place of safety for further assessment if they fulfil 3 criteria	Criteria: 1. Are in a public place, and 2. Appear to have a mental disorder, and 3. Are in immediate need of care or control	72 hours	Assessment by doctor and AMHP May lead to discharge/ informal admission/S2/S3
2 Admission for assessment Allows compulsory treatment also	Usually for first presentation of a mental disorder	28 days	Application by AMHP or NR Recommendation by 2 doctors, at least one S12 Not renewable Can be 'converted' to a S3
3 Admission for treatment Allows compulsory treatment	For known patients (usually with a firm diagnosis)	6 months	Application by AMHP or NR Recommendation by 2 doctors, at least one S12 Can be renewed: initially for 6 months, then for yearly periods
4 Emergency assessment	Shortcut when no S12 available	72 hours	Application by AMHP or NR Recommendation by any doctor Can be 'converted' to a S2
5(2) Doctor holding power for informal patients	Applies in both psychiatric and general hospitals	72 hours	Exercised by RC or deputy

Contd...

| 5(4)
Nurse holding power for informal patient | Used in the absence of an eligible doctor | 6 hours | Can be exercised by any mental health nurse
Can only lead to S5(2) or inferior status |
| 135
Assessment in private premises of a person who: appears to have a mental disorder requiring assistance and is refusing entry | Allows assessment within the premises, or removal of the person for assessment at a place of safety | N/A | Warrant required
Executing team includes doctor, AMHP and police
May lead to a S2 or S3 |

Table 13.5 Key sections of the Mental Health Act 1983 (England and Wales). AMHP, approved mental health professional; N/A, not applicable; NR, nearest relative; RC, responsible clinician; S12, Section 12 approved doctor, i.e. a doctor with particular experience in assessing and treating psychiatric conditions.

Detention under the Mental Health Act

For a patient to be detained under the MHA, the clauses below must be satisfied:

1. The person must have a mental disorder; defined by the Mental Health Act as 'any disorder or disability of the mind'. Dependence on drugs/alcohol is not considered to be a mental disorder by the Mental Health Act; nor is learning disability, unless it is 'associated with abnormally aggressive or seriously irresponsible conduct'
2. The mental disorder must be of: a nature (e.g. recurrent relapses of psychosis when without treatment), or degree (e.g. severe depression leading to self-neglect), which warrants the detention of the patient in a hospital for assessment and/or treatment
3. It must be necessary for the patient to be detained in the interests of at least one of the following: their own health (e.g. not drinking owing to psychotic depression); their own

safety (e.g. sexual disinhibition when manic); the protection of others (e.g. auditory hallucinations commanding murder)

Appropriate treatment

In addition to the above, appropriate medical treatment for the disorder must be available. Such treatment is broadly defined and includes medication, psychological treatment and rehabilitation.

Physical conditions

The MHA cannot be used to give compulsory treatment for physical conditions. If someone is deemed to lack the capacity to consent for physical treatment because of a mental condition, the Mental Capacity Act is used (see below).

Right to appeal

Patients detained under Sections 2 or 3 may appeal to a tribunal. Nearest relatives can apply to discharge a person from a Section 2 or 3 detention, although this can be barred by the responsible clinician.

Supervised community treatment

Some patients are at high risk of relapse and readmission owing to stopping their treatment after discharge ('revolving door' patients). Supervised Community treatment allows such patients to be discharged on a **community treatment order**, which means that they can be recalled to hospital if they fail to comply with certain conditions.

The Mental Capacity Act

If a person lacks capacity, they are unable to make a decision. The **Mental Capacity Act** (England and Wales) of 2005 provides legal guidance on judging capacity and making decisions on behalf of other people.

The Act states that, for a person to be judged incapable, they must be shown to have an impairment or disturbance of mental functioning, which results in them being unable to understand their condition or to make specific decisions about it.

Assessing capacity

A person lacks capacity if they are unable to perform **any** of the following:

- understand the information relevant to the decision
- retain that information
- use or weigh that information as part of the process of making the decision
- communicate their decision

Decisions made on the behalf of an incapable person must be in their best interests, and should be the least restrictive option.

Guiding principle

- A person is assumed to have capacity unless proved otherwise
- A person is not assumed to lack capacity because their decision is unwise (e.g. refusing amputation of a gangrenous leg)
- All practicable steps must be taken to help a person before judging them as lacking capacity (e.g. using a sign language interpreter for a deaf person)
- Capacity is assessed for specific decisions

Bibliography

American Psychiatric Assoication. DSM-IV-TR: Diagnostic and Statistical Manual of Mental Disorders, 4th revised edn. Arlington, VA: American Psychiatric Press; 1994.

Burton N. The Meaning of Madness. Oxford: Acheron Press; 2008.

Burton N. Clinical Skills for OSCEs, 3rd edn. Banbury: Scion Publishing; 2009.

Burton, N. Psychiatry, 2nd edn. Oxford/Chichester: Wiley-Blackwell; 2010.

David A, Fleminger S, Kopelman M, et al. Lishman's Organic Psychiatry: A Textbook of Neuropsychiatry, 4th edn. Oxford/Chichester: Wiley-Blackwell; 2009.

Fish F. Clinical Psychopathology: Signs and Symptoms in Psychiatry, 2nd edition. Bristol: John Wright & Sons Ltd; 1985.

Freud S. Mourning and Melancholia. The Standard Edition of the Complete Psychological Works of Sigmund Freud, Volume XIV (1914–1916): On the History of the Psycho-Analytic Movement, Papers on Metapsychology and Other Works. London: Hogarth Press and the Institute of Psycho-Analysis; 1953–1974: 237–258.

Gelder M, Andreason N, Lopez-Ibor J, Geddes J. New Oxford Textbook of Psychiatry, 2nd edn. Oxford: Oxford University Press; 2009.

Jamison KR. An Unquiet Mind. London: Picador; 1997.

Oyebode F. Sims' Symptoms in the Mind: An Introduction to Descriptive Psychopathology (Made Memorable), 4th edn. Edinburgh: Saunders; 2008.

Russell GFM. Bulimia nervosa: an ominous variant of anorexia nervosa. Psychol Med 1979; 9:429–48.

Szasz T. The myth of mental illness. Am Psychologist ; 1960; 15:113¬118.

Taylor D, Paton C, Kapur S. The Maudsley Prescribing Guidelines in Psychiatry, 11th edn. Oxford/Chichester: Wiley-Blackwell; 2012.

Appleby L, Nav Kapur N, Shaw J, et al. for the National Confidential Enquiry into Suicide and Homicide by People with Mental Illness. Annual Report: England, Wales and Scotland, July 2011. Manchester: The University of Manchester; 2011.

World Health Organization. ICD-10 : The ICD-10 Classification of Mental and Behavioural Disorders: Clinical Descriptions and Diagnostic Guidelines. Geneva: World Health Organization; 1992.

Index

Note: Page numbers in **bold** or *italic* refer to tables or figures respectively.